W9-ATX-717

GERIATRIC DRUG HANDBOOK

For Long-term Care

Courtesy of
McNeil Pharmaceutical
and
Ortho Pharmaceutical Corporation

GERIATRIC DRUG HANDBOOK
For Long-term Care

Jack D. McCue, M.D., F.A.C.P.
Vice Chairman, Department of Medicine
Chief, General Medicine/Geriatrics Division
Director, Medical Residency Programs
Baystate Medical Center
Springfield, Massachusetts
Professor of Medicine
Tufts University School of Medicine
Boston, Massachusetts

Edward G. Tessier, R.Ph., M.P.H., F.A.S.C.P.
Clinical Pharmacist
Baystate Medical Center
Springfield, Massachusetts 01199
Adjunct Assistant Professor of Clinical Pharmacy
Massachusetts College of Pharmacy and Allied Health Sciences
Boston, Massachusetts

Philip Gaziano, M.D.
Fellow, General Medicine/Geriatrics Division
Baystate Medical Center
Springfield, Massachusetts
Senior Clinical Fellow in Medicine
Tufts University School of Medicine
Boston, Massachusetts

Additional Contributor: Penny Lamhut, M.D.
Director, Geriatric Medical Education
Baystate Medical Center
Springfield, Massachusetts
Assistant Professor of Medicine
Tufts University School of Medicine
Boston, Massachusetts

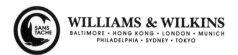

WILLIAMS & WILKINS
BALTIMORE · HONG KONG · LONDON · MUNICH
PHILADELPHIA · SYDNEY · TOKYO

Editor: Jonathan W. Pine, Jr.
Associate Editor: Carol Eckhart
Copy Editor: Shelley Potler
Designer: Wilma Rosenberger
Illustration Planner: Wayne Hubbel
Production Coordinator: Kim Nawrozki
Cover Designer: Wilma Rosenberger

Copyright © 1993
Williams & Wilkins
428 East Preston Street
Baltimore, Maryland 21202, USA

All rights reserved. This book is protected by copyright. No part of this book may be reproduced in any form or by any means, including photocopying, or utilized by any information storage and retrieval system without written permission from the copyright owner.

Accurate indications, adverse reactions, and dosage schedules for drugs are provided in this book, but it is possible that they may change. The reader is urged to review the package information data of the manufacturers of the medications mentioned.

Printed in the United States of America

Library of Congress Cataloging-in-Publication Data
McCue, Jack D.
 Geriatric drug handbook for long-term care / Jack D. McCue, Edward G. Tessier, Philip Gaziano; additional contributor, Penny Lamhut.
  p. cm.
 Includes index.
 ISBN 0-683-05793-6
 1. Geriatric pharmacology—Handbooks, manuals, etc. 2. Aged—Long-term care—Handbooks, manuals, etc. I. Tessier, Edward G.
II. Gaziano, Philip. III. Title.
RC953.7.M35 1993
618.97′061—dc20   92-23440
                                                          CIP

93 94 95 96 97
2 3 4 5 6 7 8 9 10

Introduction

This handbook is primarily designed to help physicians and other caregivers treat the approximately 1.5 million elderly, disabled Americans who live in 20,000 nursing homes in the United States. It should also be helpful to physicians who treat the independently living frail elderly (1). Nursing home admissions increase with advancing age from 14/1000 persons aged 65–74 years, to 170/1000 persons aged 85 years or more—a 1200% increase (2). At present, approximately one-half of the residents in long-term care are over 85 years old, and more than 90% of nursing home residents of any age require assistance to carry out at least one of the fundamental activities of daily living (1). In fact, the most rapidly growing segment of our population is so-called oldest-old population—a group at risk for progressive debility as a result of chronic diseases or dementia. It is predicted that the over-85-year-old segment of our population will increase at least three-fold during the half-century before the rate of growth begins to decelerate (3).

At present, nearly one-half of the population that is over 65 years old will spend some time in a nursing home (4): The average amount of time for a man over 65 years old is 0.7 years; for a woman, the average time is 1.7 years. The longer one lives, the greater the chance that one will spend some of those years in a nursing home, and the length of stay in a nursing home increases with increasing age (4).

It is not likely that medical progress will halt the growing need for nursing home care. The major cause of nursing home placement is progressive cognitive impairment, dementia, as a result of degenerative or ischemic brain disease. Persons over the age of 85 years have about a 32% risk of cognitive impairment from Alzheimer's disease; and the prevalence of dementia continues to grow with each year, with the result that significant cognitive impairment is present in the majority of 90-year-old persons and nearly universal in individuals over the age of 100 years (5). Moreover, it is probable that more, not fewer, families will be unwilling or unable to care for their elders at home in the future, increasingly turning to nursing homes for their care.

PHYSICIANS, DRUG USE, AND LONG-TERM CARE

Physicians traditionally have not been very interested in learning about or improving nursing home care. Among the many reasons for their lack of interest, one must note, is that few nursing homes have been set up to provide medical care per se: they have been designed primarily as group homes in which functionally impaired (usually aged) persons live with nursing and self-care assistance. Nurses account for about 25% of nursing home full-time equivalent (FTE) personnel and physicians account for a mere 0.3%; aides and orderlies account for 63% of FTEs (1). Only recently, as a result of intense pressures to avoid and to abbreviate hospitalizations for the elderly, nursing homes have begun to develop the types of medical services that home care agencies, such as visiting nurse associations, supply to independently living elders. Second, reimbursement for physician visits does not compensate for the inconvenience of traveling to nursing homes, especially if a physician has only a few patients there. Third, the professional satisfaction is limited: diagnostic evaluations are inconvenient, equipment is limited, there are no colleagues available to "curbside," and nursing and ancillary medical services are limited in availability and quality.

General internists and family practitioners—a shrinking group of health care providers—provide nearly all nursing home care; subspecialists have shown little interest in doing so. And until academic geriatrics was established as a quasi-subspecialty less than a decade ago, generalists had no guidance or information to help them provide care that met the needs of their nursing home patients.

Physicians who do make the effort to care for patients after admission to nursing homes tend to treat them as if they were independently living elderly patients in the office or the hospital. Unfortunately, nursing home patients really are different from independently living elderly patients—a problem that even academic geriatrics has not fully engaged, for, with some notable exceptions, academic geriatricians have not taken a great deal more interest in nursing home care than their nongeriatrician colleagues.

Nursing home patients are older, less mobile, have a variety of cognitive impairments, and suffer from multiple and often interacting chronic diseases. One result of treating nursing home patients as if they were office or hospital patients has been overmedication or, as I once called it, drug abuse of the elderly (6). Simply put, nursing home patients are treated with too many medications. They are begun on therapy without careful goal-setting, which asks why the medication is being used; therapy is continued without serious re-examination of its continuing need; dosages are too high and doses are given too frequently. As a result, the elderly nursing home patient takes, on average, eight chronically administered medications. In addition, because many nursing home patients cannot or will not tell us that they are experiencing adverse reactions, well-meaning if ill-informed drug therapy can cause deterioration in the quality of their life.

This book has a strong and, I hope, consistent point of view on drug therapy. My colleagues and I try to combine the wisdom of medical and pharmaceutical research with common sense, trying not to dodge issues and trying to give good advice when there is insufficient clinical data to give definitive recommendations. We prefer no treatment to empiric treatment unless there are clear indications for drug therapy or quality-of-life considerations dictate treatment. We prefer medications that can be given infrequently, hopefully no more than once daily, and we espouse the "start low, go slow" approach of experienced geriatricians. Because of their advanced age and chronic diseases, nursing home patients have a lower body mass, uniformly impaired renal function, and are more susceptible to adverse reactions. That knowledge informs the advice we give.

Jack D. McCue, M.D.
Springfield, MA

References

1. Hing E, Sekscenski E, Strahan GW. National Center for Health Statistics, The Nursing Home Survey. 1985 Summary for the United States. Vital and Health Statistics. Series 13, no. 97, DHHS Publ No. (PHS) 89–1758, Public Health Service, Washington, D.C. U.S. Government Printing Office, 1989.
2. Pawlson GL. Health care implications of an aging population. In: Hazzard WR, Andres R, Bierman EL, Blass JP, eds. Principles of geriatric medicine and gerontology, 2nd ed. New York: McGraw-Hill, 1990:157.

3. Besdine RW. The data base of geriatric medicine. In: Rowe JW, Besdine RW, eds. Health and disease in old age. Boston: Little, Brown, 1982:1.
4. Kemper P, Murtaugh CM. Lifetime use of nursing home care. N Engl J Med 1991;324:595.
5. White L, Cartwright W, Cornoni-Huntley J, Brock D. Geriatric epidemiology. Ann Rev Gerontol Geriatr 1986;6:215.
6. McCue JD, ed. Medical care of the elderly. Lexington, MA: Collamore Press, 1983.

Acknowledgments

Our appreciation to Linda Griffin for secretarial assistance, to Amy Marcotte, R.N., for library work, to Jack Johnson for personal inspiration and support, to Mitch Leon for invaluable advice and editorial assistance, and to our tolerant spouses.

Contents

1

Advantages of Simplicity in Long-term Care Drug Regimens

Jack D. McCue

Complicated, multiple-drug regimens are routinely prescribed for elderly residents in long-term care facilities. On average, patients in nursing homes receive six to eight medications daily (1). Potential and actual difficulties arising from multiple-drug, multiple-dose regimens include the greatly increased hazard of adverse drug reactions, the cost of medication and medical resources, detrimental effects on the quality of patients' lives, and the loss of effectiveness through drug interaction or noncompliance.

Complicated drug regimens are difficult to avoid, however, because of their tendency to "evolve" as the patient ages. Just as chronic diseases tend to accumulate and multiply with aging, so do treatments for those chronic diseases—once therapy for a chronic disease is begun, rarely is it discontinued. Only vigilant physicians will succeed at reaping the benefits of simple regimens, because few patients or nurses will question overly complex chronic drug regimens. In fact, patients and families may be puzzled by or even resist attempts to discontinue a medication that they have taken for many years, unless their physician makes special efforts to explain why a stable regimen is being changed.

HAZARDS OF COMPLEX REGIMENS

Increased Likelihood of Adverse Drug Reactions (ADRs)

The elderly may be more susceptible to ADRs than younger patients, although data are indirect (2). Lamy (3) concluded that the true incidence of ADRs is greater than that reported in the literature, which tends to deal with short-term drug reactions; it is likely that at least one-third of medications are discontinued because of an ADR and about 15–30% of hospitalizations of elderly patients are primarily because of an ADR (4).

Pharmacodynamic changes with aging are one important cause of an increase in ADRs. Changes in tissue sensitivities, such as greater central nervous system sedation with benzodiazepines, or cardiovascular changes that lead to exaggerated postural hypotension, are examples of how aging can predispose to drug toxicity (5, 6). Chronic diseases tend to magnify the incidence and severity of ADRs—hence, the elderly patient with dementia will have a more severe adverse reaction to benzodiazepines, as will the elderly hypertensive patient to cardivascular drugs.

It is most important for the physicians who care for elderly patients to know that ADRs increase, at least arithmetically, as additional drugs are added; about one-quarter of ADRs are believed to be drug-drug interactions (7–9). Jue and Vestal (10) concluded that an effort to reduce the number of drugs that elderly patients were taking resulted in a more than two-thirds reduction of the frequency of ADRs.

Decreased Quality of Life

Although one must be cautious when generalizing about the values of elderly patients, who are a more heterogeneous group both in their values and health than younger persons, older long-term care residents typically esteem the quality of their life over quantity of life more than is true of younger patients. The four major dimensions of quality of life, among the many aspects that could be examined, that seem most relevant to the elder who resides in a long-term care facility are freedom from symptoms, functional activity, psychological well-being, and cognitive function (11).

Drugs that could affect the quality of life may be grouped into two major categories. First, drugs may be used to improve the quality of life by relieving symptoms of chronic illnesses. The concern in this case is that the symptoms being treated are severe enough that the risks of the symptomatic treatment justify the chance that a serious ADR could occur. For example, tardive dyskinesia may emerge as an intractable and disfiguring complication of antipsychotic drug use for symptomatic treatment of agitation that could be treated with different drugs or without drugs, and fatal silent upper gastrointestinal bleeding may result from the use of nonsteroidal anti-inflammatory drugs (12, 13). The cognitive impairment experienced as a side effect of neurotropic drugs, such as anticonvulsants or sedatives, not only diminishes the quality of life of elders, but exposes them to the risks of hip fracture and further loss of functional independence (14, 15).

Second, drugs may be used to prevent the development or progression of chronic diseases that would lessen the quality of life. For example, many of the drugs prescribed for younger patients, such as the generally well-tolerated antihypertensive agents, trade mild side effects for a lower risk of cardiovascular disease and prolonged life expectancy; but the life expectancy for an 80-year-old patient in long-term care is probably 5 years or less, with disability increasing during the last few years of life. This is in contrast to the decades of potential benefit of antihypertensive therapy in younger persons (16). Thus, even mild side effects may justify withholding treatment for asymptomatic hypertension or diabetes (17).

Cost of Therapy

Most long-term care is paid for by patients or family, who are also responsible for the costs of drug therapy (18). Except for a few very inexpensive generic drugs, most drugs taken regularly for chronic diseases each cost $50–100 per month. There are important additional costs of drug therapy that rarely are considered by patients or physicians, however. ADRs, especially those that result in hospitalization, can be very costly. A single hospitalization for drug toxicity from generic digoxin, which usually costs less than $10 per month, can easily exceed $10,000; digoxin is a good example of an overprescribed drug that should not be administered chronically for most patients without documented rhythm disturbances.

Greater awareness of drug costs by physicians can lower the cost of prescription drugs, but the true total of drug-related costs in long-term care facilities is much more complicated than just the cost of the drug (19, 20). Most patients in long-term care have their drugs administered to them by the nursing staff; the paperwork, documentation, storage, and time devoted to administering medication and charting costs about $1 per oral dose in the acute care hospital (21); costs may be comparable in long-term care. The consequences of these additional costs are enormous for multiple-dose regimens. For example, the cost of administering inexpensive generic acetaminophen or ibuprofen four times daily in most long-term care facilities will exceed the purchase cost of the drug 5- to 10-fold.

Thus, physicians should be aware that while the costs of prescription drugs purchased by patients from community pharmacies are influenced by their highly variable mark-up pricing policies, which may unpredictably underprice or overprice drugs, they are further complicated by the costs borne by the nursing home to administer those drugs—costs that directly relate to the number of doses of drugs per day rather than to the purchase cost of the drugs. When physicians choose simpler regimens, the savings accrued from using fewer doses are gained by both the patient and the nursing home. A wisely managed nursing home will use that savings to offer more or better services to patients, or to forestall per diem rate rises, which indirectly benefits the patients.

Finally, it is important to note that while out-of-pocket expenses, such as drug therapy, are personally important to patients, drug costs overall have not risen as steeply as the other categories of medical care costs (Fig. 1.1). The growth in the costs of medical bureaucracy, for example, dwarfs that of drug costs, and the administrative costs of our cumbersome health care system now nearly equal the total costs of drug therapy (Fig. 1.2).

Lapses in Compliance

The abundant research literature and commentary on drug compliance in older patients is complicated by the variable cognitive and functional capacities of patients studied (22, 23). It seems clear, however, that elderly patients with the cognitive and functional capacity to comply with medication regimens are at least as compliant as younger patients, and probably more so (24). Chronically ill, impaired, older patients, however, are another matter. They forget to take about half of the doses of three- or four-times daily medications, they are unclear about the names or indications of many of their medications, they may double up on medications when two different doses or forms are used by the pharmacist at different times (e.g., digoxin 1 month and Lanoxin the next), and they do not report the nonprescription drugs they use when queried about their drug regimen (25–27). In short, complexity of drug

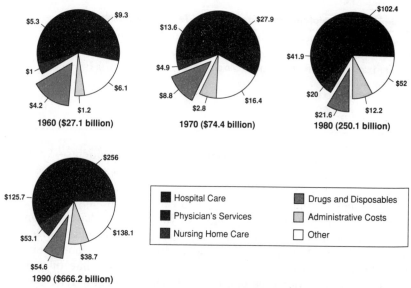

Figure 1.1. National health expenditures 1960–1990. Adapted from Iglehart JK. The American health care system. N Engl J Med 1992;326:962; and McCue JD, ed. The medical cost-containment crisis: fears, opinions, and facts. Ann Arbor: Health Administration Press, 1989.

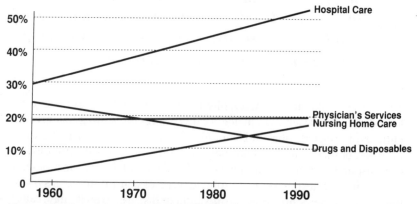

Figure 1.2. Percentage of total health care expenditure for selected years, by category of expenditure. Adapted from Iglehart JK. The American health care system. N Engl J Med 1992;326:962; and McCue JD, ed. The medical cost-containment crisis: fears, opinions, and facts. Ann Arbor: Health Administration Press, 1989.

Table 1.1. Causes of Noncompliance in Long-Term Care Facilities

Nursing error in administration
Missed doses because of absence for activities or therapy
Omitted dose because of change in clinical status
Difficulty swallowing
Refusal by confused patient
Hidden or discarded dose by patient
Unclear physician orders

regimens is the enemy of compliance for elderly outpatients—knowledge of and compliance with drug regimens decreases as the number of drugs and doses increases (28–30).

No studies of compliance in long-term care drug therapy have been published. It is probable that long-term care facilities have not only similar problems to acute-care hospitals where it is assumed that at least 5–10% of medication doses are, for a variety of reasons, not given as prescribed, but also have a unique set of problems, some of which resemble those encountered in outpatient medicine (Table 1.1). Long-term care facilities cannot usually afford highly trained nursing staff

---

. . . complexity of drug regimens is the enemy of compliance for elderly outpatients—knowledge of and compliance with drug regimens decreases as the number of drugs and doses increases.

---

around-the-clock, and primary physicians may be less responsive or more difficult to reach than in acute care settings—resulting in a greater number of transcription and administration errors. As in acute care settings, absence from the ward because of therapy, social activities, or leaves-of-absence can result in mistimed and missed doses. Most elderly patients in long-term care have some degree of central nervous system disease, e.g., dementia or cerebrovascular disease, which may cause them to refuse or to "squirrel" medication. Swallowing difficulty is common in patients with cerebrovascular disease or diabetes, and may cause problems with reliable and timely medication use.

SIMPLICITY, COMPLIANCE, AND THE PRINCIPLES OF PARSIMONY

Goal-setting is the cornerstone of rational, parsimonious drug therapy in the older, functionally impaired patient. Good communication among patient, nurses, and physician is key to goal-setting (31) (Table 1.2). The two major considerations in goal-setting that providers must keep in mind are the quality and quantity of their elderly patients' lives. For example, many 80-year-old patients, when informed that the average life expectancy of a nursing home patient in their 80s is about 5 years and that, on average, about half of those years are characterized by increasing dependence on others, would choose not to have treatment for asymptomatic conditions such as hyperlipidemia or mild to moderate hypertension, the result of which might be (statistically) a life extension of a few extra weeks. A patient in long-term care who has focal seizures but experiences significant adverse effects from anticonvulsants might prefer to risk an occasional seizure rather than continue drug therapy that results in cognitive slowing. Many conditions such as asymptomatic bacteriuria should not be treated, and others such as mild to moderate degenerative joint disease should be treated with acetaminophen for symptom relief rather than with more dangerous nonsteroidal anti-inflammatory drugs, which are unlikely to affect disease progression significantly over a 5- to 10-year period.

Every month, the physician responsible for long-term care patients should ask "Is this medication necessary?" (Table 1.3). Anticonvulsants, antianginals, antiarrhythmics, diurectics, hypnotics, psychotrop-

Table 1.2. Strategies for Improving Compliance

Communication
  Improved patient-physician communication
  Improved nurse-physician communication
Simplicity of regimens
  Preference for once-daily medications
  Eliminate all but *essential* medications
  Attention to dose formulations
Sensitivity to cognitively impaired patients
  Look for communication blocks
  All behavior makes sense, at some level

Table 1.3.   Principles of Parsimony

Before prescribing, set goals:
  Will this medication improve the quality of life?
  If not, is it *necessary*?
  If life extension is the goal, is it realistic?
Each month ask, is this medication still:
  Helpful?
  Necessary?
Use the fewest number of drugs
Use the fewest doses possible—avoid drugs with three or four daily doses
When calculating the cost of a drug, add $1 per oral *dose* for hospital or long-term care
  patients

ics, and antiarthritics can be reduced in dose or discontinued in most patients in long-term care. Typically, patients are receiving several drugs that have been started for a clinical indication that is no longer relevant—antianginals started when now-bed-to-chair patients were active and living independently, anticonvulsants started "prophylactically" for a stroke before it was known that they cause harm without benefit in the great majority of patients, antiarrhythmics started for multifocal premature ventricular contractures before it was clear that most are useless and dangerous drugs outside a critical care unit or without cardiac electrophysiological monitoring. Similarly, multiple-drug regimens are often started in acute care settings, and thereafter never seriously examined for the possibility of simplification into a single-drug regimen.

Some of the discontinued drugs may be required intermittently, and some may have to be restarted on a chronic basis. If a patient is presented with information that his or her anticonvulsant is probably resulting in some slowing of cognitive function, and if the patient has been seizure free for several years, there is a much better than 50% chance that the anticonvulsant is unnecessary; however, many will choose to attempt discontinuation. Nearly all will follow the advice of their physician when told that an attempt to withdraw drug therapy may be worthwhile.

Once-daily and twice-daily medications, e.g., antibiotics, antihypertensives, antihistamines, anti-inflammatories, are now available for most chronic and many acute diseases. In addition, most medications

Table 1.4.   Categories of Chronically Administered Drugs That Tend to be Overused in Long-term Care Facilities

Antianginal drugs
 Nitroglycerin patches and paste
 Isosorbide dinitrate
Psychotropic drugs
 Sleeping medications
 Antipsychotics in demented patients
 Antidepressants
Cardiovascular drugs
 Antiarrhythmics
 Digoxin
 Diuretics
 Antihypertensives
Anticonvulsant drugs
Laxatives and multivitamins
Nonsteroidal anti-inflammatory drugs
H_2-blockers and sucralfate

that are administered twice daily may be given once daily and those given three or four times daily to younger patients should be given no more than twice daily to older patients in long-term care (Table 1.4) Once-daily administration reduces nursing time and paperwork, increases the likelihood that a full dose of medication will be administered, decreases the chance that drug interactions will occur, reduces the frequency of gastrointestinal discomfort that occurs with each dose, and means that drug therapy is less likely to interfere with scheduled activities and treatments. For example, oral quinolones and antacids or sucralfate are incompatible because divalent metal ions bind to the fluoroquinolone molecule, preventing absorption for about 2 hours before or after the dose of the quinolone. A twice-daily quinolone such as ciprofloxacin requires a complicated dosing schedule to avoid this interaction. Substituting an H_2-antagonist would avoid the interaction, or using a longer half-life quinolone such as ofloxacin, dosed once daily in older patients with reduced renal function will reduce the window for potential drug interaction.

Table 1.4 summarizes the major categories of drugs that are excellent targets for simplification by physicians who care for patients in nursing homes—by reducing doses, by changing to single-drug regimens, or, best, by discontinuation.

References

1. Gurwitz JH, Soumerai SB, Avorn J. Improving medication prescribing and utilization in the nursing home. J Am Geriatr Soc 1990;38:542.
2. Gurwitz JH, Avorn J. The ambiguous relation between aging and adverse drug reactions. Ann Intern Med 1991;114:956.
3. Lamy PP. Adverse drug effects. Clin Geriatr Med 1990;6:293.
4. Williamson J, Chopin JM. Adverse reactions to prescribed drugs in the elderly: A multicenter investigation. Age Ageing 1980;9:73.
5. Feely J, Coakley D. Altered pharmacodynamics in the elderly. Clin Geriatr Med 1990;6:269.
6. Abernathy DR. Altered pharmacodynamics of cardiovascular drugs and their relation to altered pharmacokinetics in elderly patients. Clin Geriatr Med 1990;6:285.
7. May FE, Steward RB, Cluff LE. Drug interactions and multiple drug administration. Clin Pharmacol Ther 1977;22:322.
8. Venulet J, Blattner R, von Bulow J, et al. How good are articles on adverse drug reactions? Br Med J 1982;284.
9. Karas S. The potential for drug interactions. Ann Emerg Med 1981;10:627.
10. Jue SG, Vestal RE. Adverse drug reactions in the elderly: A critical review. In O'Malley K, ed. Medicine in old age—clinical pharmacology and drug therapy. London: Churchill Livingstone, 1985.
11. Bulpitt CJ, Fletcher AE. Drug treatment and quality of life in the elderly. Clin Geriatr Med 1990;6:309.
12. Griffin MR, Ray WA, Schaffner W. Nonsteroidal anti-inflammatory drug use and death from peptic ulcer in elderly persons. Ann Intern Med 1988;109:359.
13. Jeste DV, Wyatee RJ. Aging and tardive dyskinesia. In Miller NE, Cohen GD, eds. Schizophrenia and aging. New York: Guilford Press, 1987:275.
14. Larson EB, Kukull WA, Buchner D. Adverse drug reactions associated with global cognitive impairment in elderly persons. Ann Intern Med 1987;107:169.
15. Ray WA, Griffin MR, Schaffner W, Baugh DK, Melton LJ. Psychotropic drug use and the risk of hip fracture. N Engl J Med 1987;316:363.
16. Moritz DJ, Ostfeld AM. The epidemiology and demography of aging. Principles of gerontology, 2nd ed. New York: McGraw-Hill 1990.
17. Applegate MD. Hypertension in elderly patients. Ann Intern Med 1989;110:901.
18. Pawlson LG. Health care implications of an aging population. Principles of gerontology, 2nd ed. New York: McGraw-Hill, 1990.
19. Frazier LM, Brown JT, Divine G. Can physician education lower the cost of prescription drugs? Am Coll Phys 1991;115:116.
20. Rubinstein E, Barzilai A, Segev S, Modan M, Dickerman O, Haklai C. Antibiotic cost reduction by providing cost information. Eur J Clin Pharmacol 1988;35:269.
23. Burns E, Austin CA. Elderly patients' understanding of their drug therapy: the effect of cognitive function. Age Ageing 1990;19:236.
21. McCue JD, Tessier E. Cost containment and oral antimicrobials: issues for P&T committees. Pharmacol Toxicol 1991;334.

22. Hurd PD, Butkovich SL. Compliance problems and the older patient: assessing functional limitations. Drug Intell Clin Pharm 1986;20:228.
23. Burns E, Austin CA. Elderly patients' understanding of their drug therapy: The effect of cognitive function. Age Ageing 1990;19:236.
24. Black DM, Brand RJ, Greenlick M, et al. Compliance to treatment for hypertension in elderly patients: the SHEP pilot study. J Gerontol 1987;42:552.
25. Mahdy HA, Seymour DG. How much can elderly patients tell us about their medications? Postgrad Med J 1990;66:116.
26. Stewart RB, Caranosas GJ. Medication compliance in the elderly. Med Clin North Am 1989;73:1551.
27. Klein LE, German PS, Levine DM, et al. Medication problems among outpatients: a study with emphasis on the elderly. Ann Intern Med 1984;144:1185.
28. Eisen SA, Miller DK, Woodward RS, Spitznagel E, Przybeck TR. The effect of prescribed daily dose frequency on patient medication compliance. Arch Intern Med 1990;150:1881.
29. Helling DK, Lemke JH, Semla TP, et al. Medication use characteristics in the elderly: the Iowa 65+ rural health study. J Am Geriatr Soc 1987;35:4.
30. Greenberg RN. Overview of patient compliance with medication dosing: a literature review. Clin Ther 1984;6:592.
31. Coe RM, Prendergast CG, Psathas G. Strategies for obtaining compliance with medications regimens. J Am Geriatr Soc 1984;32:589.
32. Iglehart JK. The American health care system. N Engl J Med 1992;326:962.
33. McCue JD, ed. The medical cost-containment crisis: fears, opinions, and facts. Ann Arbor:Health Administration Press, 1989.

2
Practical Drug Use in the Elderly: Pharmacokinetic and Pharmacodynamic Considerations
Edward G. Tessier

Elderly patients living in long-term care differ from independently living elders in important ways that influence drug treatment: *(a)* they tend to be older, typically over 85 years old; *(b)* they have more chronic diseases and, hence, are more susceptible to adverse drug reactions; *(c)* most have serious cognitive deficits; *(d)* they weigh less; and *(e)* they are less mobile. In some ways, the elderly living in long-term care serve as a paradigm of the medically complicated older patient who requires the clinician's greatest skills to manage properly.

Building on a basic understanding of general pharmacokinetics (1, 2), this chapter will outline pharmacokinetic and pharmacodynamic differences noted in older patients, highlight the potential clinical significance of these differences, and provide a framework on which to base drug therapy and dosing decisions for elderly nursing home patients.

PHARMACOKINETICS

Absorption

GASTROINTESTINAL ABSORPTION

Most orally administered drugs are absorbed by passive diffusion in the small intestine. Physiological changes in the gastrointestinal tract that occur with aging and can affect the rate and/or the extent of drug absorption include a reduction in gastric acidity, diminished blood flow to the gastrointestinal tract, fewer cells through which diffusion can occur, and delayed gastric emptying (Table 2.1). In general, however, age-related changes in gastrointestinal physiology do not result in clinically important differences in drug response.

There are exceptions. Reduced gastric acidity may decrease the absorption of ketoconazole, which requires acid for conversion to

Table 2.1.   Age-Related Pharmacokinetic Differences in Absorption

Physiological Change	Impact on Pharmacokinetics	Clinical Significance
Decreased gastric acidity	Affects dissolution of drugs soluble in acid media	? Reduced absorption of ketoconazole ? Reduced effectiveness of sucralfate
Decreased gastrointestinal tract blood flow	May slow removal of drug from GI tract	Probably not clinically significant due to large surface area of small intestines, which is major site of absorption of most drugs
Fewer absorbing cells	Food and drugs may compete for absorption sites since both are generally passively diffused	May result in slowed absorption of drugs dosed with food
Delayed gastric emptying	Slow initial absorption of medication; may affect height of peak level and time to reach peak level after single dose	? Important for timing of doses of sedative hypnotics
Reduced lipid content of skin	Reduced percutaneous absorption of hydrophilic drugs	? Reduced percutaneous absorption of clonidine

hydrochloride salt prior to absorption from the stomach. Achlorhydria may also reduce the effectiveness of sucralfate, which requires hydrochloric acid to form the paste-like adhesive substance that binds to the ulcer site. Delayed gastric emptying time may retard the onset of response to drugs, clinically important in the timing of psychotropics, such as the sedative hypnotic agents.

PERCUTANEOUS ABSORPTION

The development of transdermal drug delivery systems permits the systemic delivery of low doses of certain chronically administered drugs, such as nitrates, clonidine, or opiates. There is some evidence that percutaneous or transdermal absorption of hydrophilic drugs such as clonidine is diminished in elders (3), which may be a result of the decreased lipid content of skin in elders and reduced hydration of the aging stratum corneum. Clinical significance of these observations, however, is unclear.

Distribution (Table 2.2)

CHANGES IN BODY COMPOSITION

With aging, total body water significantly decreases while total body fat increases. Total body water decreases from 70% in young adults to below 60% in men who are 70–80 years of age and below 50% in women between 70 and 80 years (4, 5). As a result, elders may have a reduced apparent volume of distribution (Vd) for water-soluble drugs, and, as such, may require lower loading doses of drugs like digoxin or aminoglycosides. Older patients are also much more likely to develop significant dehydration with aggressive diuretic use.

Body fat increases in men from about 18% in the 25-year-old to 36% in those aged 65–85 years. For women, body fat increases from 33% in 25-year-olds to 45% in 65 to 85-year-olds (5). As such, elders have a significant increase in the Vd of very fat-soluble drugs such as barbiturates, tricyclic antidepressants, and benzodiazepines. The increase in the apparent Vd of fat-soluble drugs may result in a dramatic increase in their elimination half-life. One practical result of the increases in half-life is the importance of making dosage adjustments of fat-soluble drugs slowly; it may take considerably longer to achieve steady-state concentrations of fat-soluble drugs with elders than with younger patients.

CHANGES IN SERUM PROTEINS

Alterations in plasma protein levels may affect response to drugs that bind partly or completely to plasma proteins—mostly plasma albumin for acidic drugs and α_1-acid glycoprotein for basic drugs. For highly protein-bound drugs, only a small percentage of the total serum level is unbound ("free") and available for pharmacological activity and metabolism or elimination from the body.

A modest age-related reduction in serum albumin is noted in patients

Table 2.2. Age-related Changes in Physiology That Affect Distribution of Drugs

Effect of Aging	Impact on Pharmacokinetics	Clinical Significance
↓ Body water	↓ Vd Water-soluble drugs	↓ Toxic dose threshold for digoxin, aminoglycosides; risk for dehydration with diuretic use
↑ Body fat	↑ ↑ Vd, elimination $t_{1/2}$ of fat-soluble drugs, especially for females	↑ Elimination $t_{1/2}$ benzodiazepines, tricyclic antidepressants, barbituates; allow greater period of time to achieve steady-state levels prior to dosage increases
→ ↓ Serum albumin	↑ Unbound or free drug with highly albumin-bound drugs	May affect response to phenytoin, naproxen, diazepam; ↑ risk of interactions with concurrently administered highly protein-bound drugs
→ ↓ Cardiac output	↓ Hepatic blood flow may ↓ Rate metabolism of drugs with flow-dependent metabolism	Possible ↑ response to propranolol, triazolam
→ ↓ Total body weight	↓ Mass for drug distribution	↓ Dose drugs with low therapeutic index

over the age of 70 years (6). More dramatic reductions in serum albumin are associated with hepatic and renal insufficiency, hyperthyroidism, burns, organ transplants, and malnutrition states (7), all of which may be more commonly seen in elder patients. Alternatively, infections, rheumatoid arthritis, Crohn's disease, and neoplasms are associated with increases in α_1-acid glycoprotein (25).

Patients who exhibit a marked reduction in plasma proteins may demonstrate an elevated free fraction of highly protein-bound drugs. Since many drug assays measure total serum levels (bound plus unbound), an elderly patient could have a significantly elevated free drug level and be at risk for toxicity despite a "normal" serum drug level. As Figure 2.1 illustrates, this type of phenomenon occurs with phenytoin. In general, any increase in pharmacological effect noted by an increase in free drug is short-lived as more drug is also available for distribution and metabolism/ elimination. This phenomenon may be prolonged, however, if metabolism or elimination of the drug is impaired.

DECREASED CARDIAC OUTPUT

A modest decrease in cardiac output has been attributed to aging (8), and it may be appreciably reduced in patients with heart disease. A decline in cardiac output may affect how a drug is distributed to the liver for metabolism or to the kidney for renal elimination, a clinically relevant issue for drugs for which the rate of metabolism is dependent

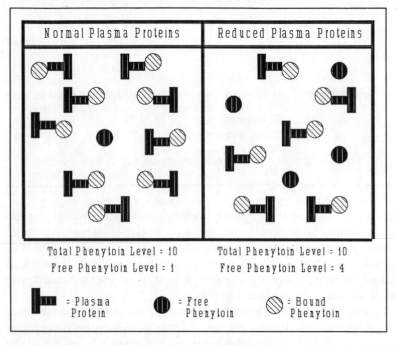

Figure 2.1. Plasma protein binding.

upon hepatic blood flow (including propranolol and triazolam). Patients who are immobile or who have circulatory disorders may also have an altered distribution profile of many drugs.

DECREASED BODY WEIGHT

Total body weight decreases linearly with age (9). Very thin, small, malnourished or dehydrated patients, typical of the chronically ill frail elderly patient in long-term care facilities, experience differences in distribution of a number of drugs as a result. Consideration of such factors as weight, hydration, and nutritional status is thus especially important when dosing drugs with a low therapeutic index (e.g., digoxin, aminoglycosides, theophylline).

Hepatic Clearance

Hepatic clearance varies among different drugs depending on chemical structure and the degree of protein binding of the drug. Patient-related influences on the rate and extent of liver metabolism of drugs include liver mass, the rate of hepatic blood flow, microsomal enzyme function, underlying liver disease, and age-associated changes in hepatic physiology. The need to change doses of medication varies greatly, however, among drug categories or even among drugs within the same category.

In general, hepatic blood flow is reduced in elders and may be markedly so in patients with a significant reduction in cardiac output. This may affect the rate of metabolism of labetalol, propranolol, and dextropropoxyphene, which exhibits a high extraction ratio (10).

The extent of plasma protein binding of a number of drugs can affect the rate of hepatic clearance by altering the amount of free drug available for metabolism. Although a modest age-related decline in plasma albumin and increase in α_1-acid glycoprotein is often observed, its clinical significance on the rate of hepatic metabolism of most drugs is unclear (11).

Liver mass is reduced 24–44% in people between the ages of 20 and 90 years (12). The reduction in liver size may explain the age-related reduction in hepatic clearance of drugs for which rate of metabolism is independent of hepatic blood flow (e.g., imipramine, theophylline) (12).

There is controversy as to whether elders exhibit a significant age-related change in microsomal (Phase I) enzyme system function

(10–12). Phase I metabolism generally results in production of more water-soluble compounds by oxidative processes. This metabolism most often occurs in the liver via cytochrome P450 enzyme systems. There is a wide inter-individual variation in the rate of cytochrome P450-mediated oxidation; this variation appears to be more related to genetic and environmental factors than to aging. Age-related differences in exposures to environmental factors (e.g., smoking, diet) may explain some differences observed in microsomal enzyme function in older individuals. Elders may have a diminished response to enzyme-inducing agents such as smoking, alcohol, and certain drugs (13), although this issue too is debated (10).

Phase II metabolism involves the conjugation reaction and usually does not involve microsomal enzyme systems. Like Phase I reactions, there appears to be significant inter-individual variation in the rate of elimination of drugs by Phase II metabolism (10). There seems to be little if any age-related change with Phase II metabolic pathways. Data for the elimination of benzodiazepines suggest that the conjugation step is unaffected by age; whether all conjugation metabolism is unaffected by age is less clear (10).

In summary, while a number of specific drugs appear to exhibit age-related changes in hepatic clearance, variation among patients in hepatic clearance is great and often unpredictable. Standard liver function tests are poor predictors of the drug-metabolizing capacity of the liver. When age-related changes in pharmacokinetic profiles of highly metabolized drugs are observed, it is difficult to determine whether the alteration is due to changes in the rate of metabolism of the drug or in differences in protein binding and/or Vd (13). The concurrent use of multiple hepatically cleared drugs, however, may strain the limited reserve capacity of the aging liver, slowing the rate of metabolism of one or more of the drugs. Drugs with potentially clinically significant age-related alterations in hepatic metabolism are listed in Table 2.3.

Renal Elimination

Renal mass, renal blood flow, and the number of functioning glomeruli all decline with age (14). It is, therefore, not surprising that glomerular filtration rate (GFR) as measured by creatinine clearance declines with age (14, 15). Interestingly, for reasons that are not clear,

Table 2.3.   Drugs Exhibiting Age-Related Reductions in Hepatic Clearance[a]

Agent	Proposed Mechanism
Dextropropoxyphene	? Hepatic blood flow
Amitriptyline, desipramine, imipramine, nortriptyline	? ↓ Hepatic mass
Chlordiazepoxide, diazepam, flurazepam	? Changes in microsomal enzyme function; ? ↓ hepatic mass
? Lidocaine	? Hepatic blood flow; ? volume of distribution? (variation in study results)
? Theophylline	? ↓ Hepatic mass. (wide variation in study results; significant age-related differences most often noted in non-smokers)
Labetalol, ? Propranolol	? Hepatic blood flow. (variation in study results)

[a]Adapted from Durnas C, Loi CM, Cusack BJ. Hepatic drug metabolism and aging. Appendix. Clin Pharmacokinet 1990;19:359.

a significant number of elder patients (up to one-third) demonstrate little or no age-related renal insufficiency (14, 16). The great majority of patients, those who demonstrate a decline in renal function, can experience accumulation of drugs that are eliminated by the kidney as either unchanged drug or active metabolites. Table 2.4 is a partial list of drugs that must be used cautiously and/or require dosage adjustment in patients with reduced renal function.

An accurate assessment of renal function is helpful when dosing all renally excreted drugs, and it is essential for those renally eliminated drugs with a low therapeutic index, such as digoxin, theophylline, or aminoglycosides. Unfortunately, serum creatinine and blood urea nitro-

An accurate assessment of renal function is helpful when dosing all renally excreted drugs, and it is essential for those renally eliminated . . .

Table 2.4.   Drugs Requiring Dosage Adjustment and/or Cautious Use in Patients with Renal Insufficiency[a]

Antimicrobials:	Cardiovascular Drugs
Aminoglycosides[b]	ACE-inhibitors[c]
Ampicillin[b]	β-Adrenoceptor blockers
Amoxicillin[b]	Acebutolol[b]
Aztreonam[b]	Atenolol[b]
Cefazolin[b]	Nadolol[b]
Ceftazidime[b]	Amiloride[b,c]
Ceftizoxime[b]	Digoxin[b]
Cephradine[b]	Disopyramide[b]
Ciprofloxacin[b]	Methyldopa[b]
Fluconazole[b]	Procainamide[b]
Imipenem/cilastatin[b]	Thiazide diuretics[c]
Lomefloxacin[b]	
Metronidazole[b]	Gastrointestinal Drugs
Mezlocillin[b]	Cimetidine[b]
Nitrofurantoin[c]	Famotidine[b]
Ofloxacin[b]	Metoclopramide[b]
Sulfamethoxazole/trimethoprim[b]	Ranitidine[b]
Tetracycline[c]	
Ticarcillin[b]	Nonsteroidal Anti-Inflammatory Agents[c]
Vancomycin[b]	
	Miscellaneous
Antivirals	Allopurinol[b]
Acyclovir[b]	Chlorpropamide[c]
Amantadine[b]	Clofibrate[b]
	Diphenhydramine[b]
	Ethambutol[b]
	Insulin[b]
	Lithium carbonate[b,c]
	Quinine sulfate[b]

[a] Adapted from Bennett WM. Guide to drug dosage in renal failure. Clin Pharmacokinet 1988;15:326.
[b] Indicates dosage adjustment may be required.
[c] Should be avoided in patients with significant renal insufficiency.

gen levels alone are insufficient to estimate the extent of renal compromise in many older patients. Blood urea nitrogen levels are not specific indicators of renal function and may be affected by protein intake, hydration status, hepatic function, and bowel flora. Serum creatinine levels are related to both muscle mass and renal function. Older patients have reduced muscle mass and produce less creatinine;

hence, an older patient with a "normal" serum creatinine of 1.0 g/dl may, in fact, have significant renal impairment, with a creatinine clearance less than 30% of normal.

Creatinine clearance is a more accurate measure of renal function in older patients. While obtaining a 24-hour urine creatinine clearance, which may require an indwelling catheter for 24 hours, may be appropriate if an accurate assessment of renal function is required, a "ballpark" creatinine clearance can be easily and fairly reliably estimated utilizing the Cockcroft and Gault formula (17–20). Alternatively, the Jelliffe formula provides a means to estimate creatinine clearance in the absence of weight, but was originally intended for patients under 80 years of age (21) (Fig. 2.2). Correct calculation of the creatinine clearance estimates requires that the serum creatinine be at a steady state and should ideally be drawn in the fasting state.

These formulae may overestimate renal function by as much as 40% in patients who have extraordinarily reduced muscle mass or are immobile (17), but considerable underestimation has also been observed with such patients (22, 23)—important considerations for many long-term care patients. For such patients, careful interpretation of creatinine

Cockcroft and Gault Formula (17):

$$\text{Males: } \frac{(140 - \text{age}) \ (\text{Lean Body Wt in kg})}{(72)(\text{Serum Creatinine})}$$

$$\text{Females: } \frac{(0.85) \times (140 - \text{age}) \ (\text{Lean Body Wt in kg})}{(72) \ (\text{Serum Creatinine})}$$

Lean Body Weight:
  Males: 50 kg + 2.3 kg for each inch over 5 feet
  Females: 45 kg + 2.3 kg for each inch over 5 feet

Jelliffe Formula (21):

$$\text{Males: } \frac{98 - [(0.8) \ (\text{Age} - 20)]}{\text{Serum Creatinine}}$$

$$\text{Females: } \frac{(0.9) \times 98 - [(0.8) \ (\text{Age} - 20)]}{\text{Serum Creatinine}}$$

Figure 2.2.   Estimating renal function.

clearance estimates is required. Estimates of creatinine clearance do not eliminate the need to obtain appropriately timed drug levels of potentially toxic, renally excreted drugs (e.g., aminoglycosides) (24).

PHARMACODYNAMICS

General Principles

Age-related changes in an individual patient's anatomy and physiology may result in an altered *response* to drugs that can be independent of, or in addition to, changes in drug concentration at the receptor site(s). The general term for how individual patients respond to drugs is pharmacodynamics—a concept of growing importance for those who take care of elderly patients.

Homeostatic reserve is reduced with age. Thus, the elder patient's ability to respond to changes in the environment or to physiological challenges such as acute illness may be impaired. Changes in receptor site density, characteristics of the receptor site, or changes in the processes by which the activated receptor transduces the signal in part explain age-related pharmacodynamic changes observed with many drugs (25). Pharmacodynamic changes with aging are much more likely to result in clinically important drug reactions than the pharmacokinetic changes previously described. Drugs exhibiting age-related changes in pharmacodynamic parameters are listed in Table 2.5.

Some examples of pharmacodynamic changes that result in potentially hazardous adverse drug reactions are:

1. The maintenance of upright position in elders requires increases in the frequency and amplitude of corrective movements, which may be related to age-associated reduction in dopamine receptors in the striatum (25). Sedatives appear to impair corrective mechanisms and may be an explanation for the increased frequency of falls associated with sedative-hypnotic use in elder patients.
2. Ability to maintain blood pressure during postural changes is impaired in the elderly. This loss of homeostatic reserve can often result in symptomatic positional or orthostatic hypotension; the effect may be accentuated with drugs associated with hypotensive responses, α-adrenergic blocking agents and agents that reduce sympa-

Table 2.5. Clinically Significant Age-Related Changes in Pharmacodynamic Response[a]

Adverse Clinical Event	Drug	Age-related Mechanism of Change
Falls	Sedative-hypnotics	Impaired mechanism of maintaining postural control
	Antihypertensives	Vasodilation
	Tricyclic antidepressants	α-Adrenergic blockade
	Neuroleptics	Reduced baroreceptor activity
	Diuretics	Volume depletion
Reduced intestinal motility Constipation Impaction Intestinal obstruction	Anticholinergics Tricyclic antidepressants Antihistamines	Anticholinergic effects
Disorientation Delirium Psychosis	Anticholinergics Tricyclic antidepressants Antihistamines	Anticholinergic effects
	Benzodiazepines	↑ Benzodiazepine receptor sensitivity
	Amphetamines Theophylline β-Agonists Levodopa	CNS stimulation
Urinary incontinence	Diuretics	Bladder filling exceeds capacity
	Anticholinergics Tricyclic antidepressants Antihistamines	Urinary outflow obstruction (especially males with BPH)
Edema, worsening CHF	Corticosteroids Saline laxatives/enemas	Sodium retention
Tardive dyskinesia Extrapyramidal symptoms	Neuroleptics Metoclopramide	Depletion of CNS dopamine
↓ Response to Pharmacotherapy	β-Adrenergic blockers β-Adrenergic agonists	↓ β-Adrenergic receptor site function or transduction ↓ β-Adrenergic receptors ↓ Affinity for receptor site
	Clonidine Prazosin	↓ α_2-Adrenergic receptor responsiveness

Table 2.5.   Clinically Significant Age-Related Changes in Pharmacodynamic Response[a] **Continued**

Adverse Clinical Event	Drug	Age-related Mechanism of Change
↑ Response to pharmacotherapy	Benzodiazepines Warfarin	↑ Benzodiazepine receptor sensitivity ↑ Anticoagulant effect at same dose (? Vitamin K dependent?)
Hyperglycemia	Thiazide diuretics β-Adrenergic blockers Corticosteroids	↓ Glucose tolerance

[a]Adapted, in part, from Swift CG. Pharmacodynamics: changes in homeostatic mechanisms, receptor and target organ sensitivity in the elderly. Br Med Bull 1990;46:36.

thetic outflow from the central nervous system (CNS), resulting in falling or dizziness with postural movements.

3. Intestinal motility declines with age and immobility. Hence, drugs with anticholinergic effects are particularly problematic in nursing home patients, resulting in constipation or even intestinal obstruction.

4. Elderly men with urinary outflow obstruction frequently develop urinary retention when taking anticholinergic agents. Alternatively, patients with bladder instability develop urinary incontinence when given diuretics because urine flow quickly exceeds their bladder capacity (25).

5. Memory and orientation in the elderly are more sensitive to impairment by sedative agents, CNS stimulants, and anticholinergic agents (26). Thus, a low dose of a benzodiazepine will result in more confusion in an elderly person than a higher dose in a younger person, who may experience only sedation with no cognitive disturbance.

6. Elders appear to have a reduced response at both the β-adrenergic and α_1-adrenergic receptor sites. Clinical implications for the therapeutic response to β-adrenergic blockers, and α_2-adrenergic blockers may be significant. For example, β-adrenergic blockers result in lessened or no bradycardic response in the elderly, resulting in excessive dosing by clinicians who use pulse rate to assess the adequacy of β-blocker regimens.

7. Elders appear to be more sensitive to the sedative effects of benzodiazepines after initial dosing, an effect that cannot be explained by age-associated pharmacokinetic differences alone. Similar age-related alterations in response to calcium channel-blockers and warfarin (27) are also observed.

GENERAL PRINCIPLES IN DRUG THERAPY AND DOSING

Age-related physiological changes affect the pharmacokinetic and pharmacodynamic profiles of a large number of drugs and predispose elders to significant drug toxicity. While there is considerable variation in how elders respond to drug therapy, a number of general principles can be applied to instituting or adjusting drug therapy with older patients.

1. *Set treatment goals: establish and document a clear indication and determine the necessity of initiating drug therapy.*
2. *Identify underlying disease states that may alter drug response.* Especially important are chronic diseases that alter the pharmacokinetics and pharmacodynamic response to drugs, (e.g., congestive heart failure, chronic renal failure).
3. *Obtain an accurate past drug history.* Consider drug allergies, prior sensitivities, and include over-the-counter and p.r.n. medications.
4. *Obtain baseline:*
   Orthostatic blood pressures: especially important if utilizing diuretics, antihypertensives, tricyclic antidepressants;
   Cognitive function assessments: especially important for drugs with anticholinergic and sedative effects;
   Bowel function and urinary tract function assessments: especially important for drugs with anticholinergic effects.
5. *Establish a baseline of minimal data necessary for appropriate dosing.* Include:
   Total body weight;
   Height (in establishing lean body weight);
   Serum creatinine and estimated or actual creatinine clearance;
   Albumin (if utilizing highly protein-bound drugs or suspect altered drug response may be related to altered protein binding).

6. *Whenever possible, start with low doses and make dosage adjustments slowly.* This is especially important for lipophilic drugs such as benzodiazepines, barbiturates, and tricyclic antidepressants that may require an extended period of time to reach steady-state serum levels after dosage adjustment.
7. *Recognize wide interpatient variability in drug response.*
8. *Simplify the drug regimen.* Carefully consider the risk and benefit of every medication the patient receives. Simplified regimens reduce the risk for negative outcomes, reduce patient cost, and increase patient compliance.
9. *Establish open communication with the patient, family, and/or nursing staff in assessing response to drug therapy.*

References

1. Evans WE, Schentag JJ, Jusko WJ, eds. Applied pharmacokinetics: principles of therapeutic drug monitoring, 2nd Ed. Spokane, WA: Applied Therapeutics, Inc. 1986.
2. Winter ME. Basic clinical pharmacokinetics, 2nd Ed. Vancouver, WA: Applied Therapeutics, Inc. 1988.
3. Roskos KV, Maibach HI, Guy RH. The effect of aging on percutaneous absorption in man. J Pharmacokinet Biopharm 1989;17:617.
4. Schoeller DA. Changes in total body water with age. Am J Clin Nutr 1989;50:1176.
5. Kuczmarski RJ. Need for body composition information in elderly subjects. Am J Clin Nutr 1989;50:1150.
6. Cooper JK, Gardner C. Effect of aging on serum albumin. J Am Geriatr Soc 1989;37:1039.
7. Zini R, Riant P, Barre J, Tillement JP. Disease-induced variations in plasma protein levels—implications for drug dosage regimens, Parts 1 & 2. Clin Pharmacokinet 1990;19:147, 218.
8. Safar M. Ageing and its effects on the cardiovascular system. Drugs 1990;39:(Suppl 1):1.
9. Master AM, Lasser RP, Beckman G. Tables of average weight and height of Americans aged 65 to 94 years. JAMA 1960;172:659.
10. Durnas C, Loi CM, Cusack BJ. Hepatic drug metabolism and aging. Clin Pharmacokinet 1990;19:359.
11. Vestal RE. Aging and determents of hepatic drug clearance. Hepatology 1989;9:331.
12. Woodhouse KW, James OFW, Hepatic drug metabolism and aging. Br Med Bull 1990;46:22.
13. Tsujimoto G, Hashimoto K, Hoffman BB. Pharmacokinetic and pharmacodynamic principles of drug therapy in old age—part 1. Int J Clin Pharmacol Ther Toxicol 1989;27:13.

14. Roy AT, Johnson LE, Lee DB, et al. Renal failure in older people—UCLA grand rounds. J Am Geriatr Soc 1990;38:239.
15. Danziger RS, Tobin JD, Becker LC, et al. The age-associated decline in glomerular filtration in healthy normotensive volunteers—Lack of relationship to cardiovascular performance. J Am Geriatr Soc 1990;38:1127.
16. Bennett WM. Geriatric pharmacokinetics and the kidney. Am J Kidney Dis 1990;16:283.
17. Cockcroft DW, Gault MH. Prediction of creatinine clearance from serum creatinine. Nephron 1976;16:31.
18. Durakovic Z. Creatinine clearance in the elderly: a comparison of direct measurement and calculation from serum creatinine. Nephron 1986;44:66.
19. Beck CL, Pucino F, Carlson JD, et al. Evaluation of creatinine clearance estimation in an elderly male population. Pharmacotherapy 1988;8:183.
20. O'Connell MB, Dwinell AM, Bannick-Mohrland SD. Predictive performance of equations to estimate creatinine clearance in hospitalized elderly patients. DICP Ann Pharmacother 1992;26:627.
21. Jelliffe RW. Creatinine clearance: bedside estimate. Ann Intern Med 1973;79:604.
22. Drinka PJ. Estimating creatinine clearance from serum creatinine in chronically immobilized nursing home residents. Nephron 1987;47:310.
23. Drusano GL, Muncie HL, Hoopes JM, et al. Commonly used methods of estimating creatinine clearance are inadequate for elderly debilitated nursing home patients. J Am Geriatr Soc 1988;36:437.
24. Goldberg TH, Finkelstein MS. Difficulties in estimating glomerular filtration rate in the elderly. Arch Intern Med 1987;147:1430.
25. Swift CG. Pharmacodynamics: changes in homeostatic mechanisms, receptor and target organ sensitivity in the elderly. Br Med Bull 1990;46:36.
26. Ray PG, Meador KJ, Loring DW, et al. Central anticholinergic hypersensitivity in aging. J Geriatr Psychiatry Neurol 1992;5:72.
27. Gurwitz JH, Avorn J, Ross-Degnan D, et al. Aging and the anticoagulant response to warfarin therapy. Ann Intern Med 1992;116:901.

3

Antibiotic Selection in Long-term Care

Jack D. McCue

The pathogens that cause infections in nursing homes have typically been characterized as bacteriologically intermediate between community-acquired and hospital-acquired infections. While this characterization is useful to help clinicians recognize that the spectrum of pathogens and the complexity of infections in long-term care differs from those encountered in the infections of community-living elders, it is an oversimplification.

The only accurate generalization about nursing homes is that they, like hospitals, are ecologically individual—they are bacteriologically unique, dynamic environments. Their ecology is a reflection of the types of organisms that colonize patients who are transferred from acute care settings (all of which have their own microbiologically peculiar environments) plus the types of organisms that are encountered in community-acquired infections; but just as hospitals evolve their own ecology as a result of antibiotic selection in their intensive care units, the types of patients treated, and their physicians' customary antibiotic usage patterns, so do nursing homes. Hence, staphylococcal or *Pseudomonas* infections may be common in some long-term care facilities, and rare in others; antibiotic resistance in common enterobacteriaceae such as *Escherichia coli* may be a negligible problem in some facilities, and others may have to contend with widespread antibiotic resistance problems like methicillin-resistant or ciprofloxacin-resistant staphylococci—similar to resistance patterns encountered in intensive care units in different hospitals (1, 2).

Moreover, the types of patients who get infections in nursing homes are different. Serious infections afflict the relatively healthy as well as the debilitated elderly more often, causing excess morbidity and mortality in comparison with younger patients, but there is no doubt that the debilitated, chronically ill elder is at greater risk for frequent, severe, and complicated infections (3–5) (Table 3.1). Overall, mortality attributable to infection is two to ten times greater for elderly hospitalized patients compared with younger patients (4); much, but not all of the increased mortality can be attributed to the severity of underlying

Table 3.1.   Categories of Elderly Patients Requiring Consideration of Altered Antibiotic Dosing Regimens

All patients over 80 years old
Frail elderly (low body weight and multiple chronic diseases)
Serum creatinine >1.0 mg/dl
Immobile patients with reduced muscle mass
Patients taking multiple drugs, especially
   Anticonvulsants
   Antacids and H_2-antagonists
   Theophylline
   Anticoagulants

diseases, such as cancer, chronic lung disease, or renal failure (6). Poor outcome of treatment in elderly patients, however, is also a result of delays in treatment—in part a result of atypical presentations of serious bacterial infections, a higher prevalence of adverse reactions to antimicrobial agents, and inattention to clinically contributing factors such as poor cough, incomplete bladder emptying, or poor nutrition.

TYPES OF INFECTIONS

Important causes of bacterial infections in the elderly and some of the clinically relevant differences from infections in younger patients are summarized in Table 3.2. The causes of more than 80% of infections in long-term care are urinary tract infections (UTIs), lower respiratory infections, and soft tissue infections related to pressure sores (7–10). This knowledge greatly simplifies the diagnostic approach of the clinician. A chest examination, visual examination of the urine [cloudiness usually indicates more than 50 white blood cells (WBCs) per high-powered field (HPF) on urinalysis], abdominal palpation, and skin

The causes of more than 80% of infections in long-term care are urinary tract infections (UTIs), lower respiratory infections, and soft tissue infections related to pressure sores.

Table 3.2.   Important Categories of Infections in the Elderly Long-term Care Patient[a]

Category	Clinical Comments	Empiric Regimens

Urinary tract infections	Most common cause of infection and bacteremia in LTC patients; bladder dysfunction or obstruction universal; highly antibiotic-resistant pathogens are uncommon without indwelling catheter; treat for at least 7 days; asymptomatic bacteriuria or bacteriuria without pyuria should not usually be treated	Oral
		  Trimethoprim-sulfamethoxazole 2 DS tabs b.i.d.
		  Ofloxacin (Floxin) 200 mg b.i.d.
		  Cefixime (Suprax) 400 mg qday
		Parenteral
		  A third-generation cephalosporin (IM/IV)

Respiratory infections	Reliable sputum specimens not obtainable from most patients; distinction among exacerbation of chronic bronchitis, aspiration, and pneumonia of limited utility; *Pneumococcus* is relatively uncommon; polymicrobial infections are common; empiric therapy should be broad.	Oral
		  Ofloxacin (Floxin) 400 mg b.i.d.
		  Cefixime (Suprax) 400 mg qday
		Parenteral
		  A third-generation cephalosporin (IM/IV)
		  Quinolone (IV)

Abdominal infections	Empyema of gallbladder or acute cholecystitis, periappendiceal or diverticular abscess, *C. difficile* and other enteric infections, and cancer-related infections more common	Oral
		  Amoxicillin-clavulanate (Augmentin) 500 mg t.i.d.
		  Metronidazole (Flagyl) 500 mg b.i.d. and ofloxacin (Floxin) 400 mg b.i.d.
		Parenteral
		  Cefotetan (Cefotan) 1 g b.i.d. (IM/IV)

examination for cellulitis will reveal the cause of infection or exclude serious bacterial infection in nearly all febrile nursing home patients; only a small minority of patients will require more in-depth investigations for a source of infection.

The characteristics of the infections encountered in long-term care patients are different as well. Short-course therapy for UTIs yields poor

Table 3.2. Important Categories of Infections in the Elderly Long-term Care Patient[a] Continued

Category	Clinical Comments	Empiric Regimens
Soft-tissue infections	Typically polymicrobial and associated with pressure sores, skin tears, or vascular insufficiency; role of anaerobic bacteria exaggerated; underlying osteomyelitis frequently missed by clinicians; utility of broad- versus narrow-spectrum treatment not well defined	Oral 　Ofloxacin (Floxin) 400 mg b.i.d. 　Amoxicillin-clavulanate 　(Augmentin) 250 mg t.i.d. Parenteral 　A cephalosporin (IM/IV) 　Quinolone (IV)
Fever of Unknown Origin	Consider osteomyelitis, drug fever (especially TMP/SMX), infective endocarditis, chronic aspiration, gallbladder disease, septic arthritis, and tuberculosis	

[a]Dosing is based on treatment recommendations for a moderately seriously infected 55-kg 80-year-old patient with a serum creatinine of 1.2 mg% (calculated creatinine clearance approximately 30 ml/min).

long-term bacterial eradication (11); because nearly all UTIs of the elderly are complicated by bladder dysfunction, obstruction, or chronic catheterization, 10–14 days of therapy is prudent—rather than the 1- to 3-day therapy that gives good results in younger patients. Aspiration must be suspected as a cause of all respiratory infections, making [*Streptococcus pneumoniae*] a less common pathogen. Soft tissue infections are more complicated because trauma, pressure, or vascular insufficiency must be assumed to be possible contributing factors. Viral infections, with the exception of influenza, are infrequent causes of fever because nursing home patients are an ecologically isolated population, and rarely come in contact with children who are important vectors in the transmission of viral infections.

Most elderly patients with serious bacterial infections are febrile, but up to one-third of debilitated elderly patients with bacterial infections such as pneumonia or bacteremic UTI will not be febrile at the time of initial evaluation, because of a disordered thermoregulatory response or deficient host defenses (12–18). On the other hand, fever exceeding 101°F reliably indicates a high probability of bacterial infection (19). The presenting symptoms of patients with no fever or low-grade fever who have bacterial infection are most commonly alterations in mental status. These may be as subtle as unwillingness to interact with caregivers or to participate in self-care, loss of interest in eating, confusion, falls, incontinence, chest pain, or refusal to drink. For example, a study of elderly men with pneumonia found that only one-third had cough and fever, and 10% had no symptom suggestive of pneumonia (20).

PRINCIPLES OF ANTIBIOTIC THERAPY IN THE NURSING HOME

1. Empiric therapy should be broad in spectrum and should be administered early. Narrow-spectrum therapy, such as oral penicillins or limited-spectrum cephalosporins, should be used only for the treatment of defined infections. Other infections should be initially assumed to be caused by a wide range of potential pathogens including enteric gram-negative bacilli, staphylococci, and, in some cases, anaerobic bacteria.
2. Parenteral therapy, if required, should be changed to oral therapy as soon as the nature of the infection is defined and the acute symptoms and signs have abated.
3. Multiple-drug parenteral regimens are very rarely necessary, are more costly, increase the risk of adverse drug reactions, and do not improve outcome when compared with an appropriate single-drug antimicrobial regimen.
4. Aminoglycosides should not be used and are almost never needed. Parenteral cephalosporins and quinolones, and oral quinolones have a spectrum of activity among gram-negative bacilli and are much safer.
5. Dosing should assume that very elderly patients without recognized renal disease have a creatinine clearance of about 50 ml/min; dose intervals should be increased. For example, among the quinolones, a variety of dosing changes are recommended for a patient with a creatinine clearance of 40–50 ml/min: ciprofloxacin is given q18h and ofloxacin is given once daily.
6. Pharmacokinetics of IM administration are comparable to IV administration for nearly all antibiotics that can be given IM. IM antibiotics

may be used safely in patients who are not hypotensive and who cannot take oral therapy.

7. Oral regimens are well-absorbed, reliable therapy in elderly patients, and are preferred to IM or IV regimens.

EMPIRIC REGIMENS

As summarized in Table 3.3, oral antimicrobials can be divided into broad-spectrum agents that are useful for empiric therapy of the major causes of bacterial infection in long-term care facilities and narrow-spectrum agents that should be used only for defined infectious diseases. Antimicrobials with an established once- or twice-daily dosing regimen and a low side-effect profile are preferentially listed.

Table 3.4 summarizes parenteral antibiotics suitable for empiric therapy of serious infections that can also be administered IM—cephalosporins and, more recently, imipenem/cilastatin. Some patients tolerate intramuscular cephalosporins without discomfort, while others appreciate the addition of lidocaine to the injection. Only a small minority of nursing homes can administer intravenous therapy; if so, the broad-spectrum penicillins, such as mezlocillin, piperacillin, or ticarcillin/clavulanate are also potentially useful for empiric therapy of presumed gram-negative bacillary (***), streptococcal (***), respiratory pathogen (***), anaerobic (***), or resistant gram-negative bacillary infection (**) (see Table 4.3 for key). Only ticarcillin/clavulanate has antistaphylococcal activity (**). The penicillins cannot be given IM in full doses for empiric therapy of serious infections.

The remarkable bioavailability of the new quinolones, like ofloxacin, makes parenteral administration unnecessary for patients who can take medications by mouth. Ciprofloxacin (at reduced doses) and ofloxacin (at the same doses as for oral therapy because of its oral-intravenous bioequivalence) may be administered IV, but not IM. A potential advantage to the empiric use of parenteral quinolone therapy is the simplicity of step-down therapy to definitive bioequivalent oral regimens—which is not true for any of the cephalosporins, penicillins, or other β-lactam antibiotics (21, 22).

An abbreviated listing of recommendations for empiric regimens for the major causes of infections in long-term care is given in Table 3.2.

Table 3.3. Selected Oral Antimicrobials Useful in Long-term Care[a]

Drug	Usual Full Dose	Usual Half-Life	ESRD† Half-Life	Frail Elder Dose††	Strepto-cocci	Staphylo-cocci	Community-acquired Gram-negative Activity	Respiratory Pathogen Activity	Anaerobe Activity	Hospital-acquired Gram-negative Activity
Penicillin V	500 mg q6h	0.5h	6–20h	250 mg q8h	***	0	0	*	*	0
Dicloxacillin	500 mg q6h	0.6–0.8h	6–20h	250 mg q8h	**	***	0	*	*	0
Amoxicillin	500 mg q8h	1.0–1.2h	7.5–20.0h	250 mg q8h	***	0	*	**	*	0
Amoxicillin-clavulanate	500 mg q8h	1.0–1.2h	7.5–20.0h	250 mg q8h	***	**	**	***	***	*
Cefuroxime-axetil	500 mg q12h	1–2h	15–20h	250 mg q12h	***	***	**	***	*	0
Cefixime	400 mg qday	2.4–4.0h	12h	200–400 mg qday	***	0	**	***	*	*
Cotrimoxazole	1 DS q12h	8–13h	>26h	1 reg tab q12h	***	**	***	***	0	*

Antibiotic	Dose	$t_{1/2}$	$t_{1/2}$ ESRD	Frail Elder Dose	Activity[a]					
Ciprofloxacin	500 mg q12h	3.0–4.8h	4.4–12.6h	250 mg q12h	*	***	***	***	*	***
Ofloxacin	400 mg q12h	4.9–6.9h	16.9–28.4h	200 mg q24h	**	***	***	***	*	***
Metronidazole	500 mg q8–12h	6–8h	6–8h	500 mg q8–12h	0	0	0	0	***	0
Clindamycin	300 mg q6–8h	2–3h	3–4h	300 mg q8h	***	***	0	*	***	0
Clarithromycin	500 mg q12h	5–7h	15–50h	250 mg q12h	***	***	0	***	*	0
Azithromycin	250 mg q24h	48h	48h	250 mg q24h	***	***	0	***	*	0
Erythromycin	500 mg q6h	1.5–2.0h	6h	250 mg q8h	***	***	0	**	*	0

aAntibacterial activity (see Table 3.2):
0—not active;
*—some activity;
**—moderate activity;
***—highly active.

ESRD†—end stage renal disease
Frail Elder Dose††—typical dose for a 50–60kg, 80 year old woman with a serum creatinine of 1.0mg percent

Table 3.4. Selected Parenteral Antimicrobials Useful in Long-term Care (IV/IM Administration)[a]

Antimicrobial	Typical Dose	Streptococci	Staphylococci	Gram-negative Bacilli	Resistant Gram-negative Bacilli	Respiratory Pathogens	Anaerobes
Cefazolin (Ancef/Kefzol)	1 g q12h	***	***	**	*	*	*
Cefotetan (Cefotan)	1 g q12h	***	***	***	*	**	***
Ceftrianxone (Rocephin)	1 g q12h	***	**	***	**	***	*
Ceftazidime (Fortaz) or Cefoperazone (Cefobid)	1 g q12h	***	**	***	***	***	*
Imipenem/cilastatin (Primaxin)	500 mg q12h	***	**	***	**	***	***
Ofloxacin (IV only) (Floxin)	400 mg q12h	**	***	***	**	***	*

[a]Useful antibacterial activity (0 to ***).

Urinary Tract Infections

Asymptomatic bacteriuria is common in elderly nursing home patients and, as a result, fever or nonspecific indicators of infection may be misattributed to UTI (23). Patients do not benefit from treatment of asymptomatic bacteriuria, although the presence of symptoms may be hard to determine in patients with cognitive deficits, and most clinicians would treat asymptomatic bacteriuria that is accompanied by significant pyuria (24, 25).

Rarely do UTIs require parenteral therapy unless the patient is unable to take oral medications. Trimethoprim-sulfamethoxazole or co-trimoxazole (TMP/SMX), β-lactam antibiotics, and quinolones are present in high concentrations in urine, and are the preferred oral therapy. Broad-spectrum agents should be chosen: TMP/SMX and quinolones give superior cure rates to β-lactam antimicrobials in short-course regimens for uncomplicated UTI. In complicated UTI, however, quinolones are clinically superior to other regimens including TMP/SMX, but are probably equivalent in 10-day regimens. All of the fluoroquinolone antimicrobials except norfloxacin probably give equivalent results, although ofloxacin has been tested more extensively in the elderly, usually in twice-daily regimens.

In conflict with the prescribing habits of many nursing home clinicians, limited-spectrum cephalosporins and penicillins (cephalexin, cefaclor, amoxicillin) are poor choices for empiric therapy of complicated UTI. Cefixime and amoxicillin-clavulanate, and cefuroxime axetil to a lesser extent, are the only oral β-lactam antibiotics with a sufficiently broad spectrum of activity to justify empiric use. A new oral cephalosporin, cefprozil, has similar antibacterial activity to cefaclor, but improved pharmacokinetics, thereby allowing less frequent dosing (26).

Two new macrolide antibiotics, clarithromycin and azithromycin (27), have not been studied extensively in the elderly. They are, however, promising drugs that are more active in vitro, have broader spectra of activity, superior pharmacokinetics, and fewer gastrointestinal (GI) side effects than erythromycin.

The third-generation cephalosporins have a broader spectrum of activity, some have a prolonged half-life, and do not differ greatly in costs when given in geriatric IM doses. Typical IM/IV regimens (Table

3.3) for seriously ill or potentially bacteremic patients are ceftriaxone, 1 g qday; ceftazidime, 1 g q12h; cefoperazone, 1 g q12h; imipenem/ cilastatin, 500 mg q12h; or IV-only ofloxacin, 400 mg q12h; and mezlocillin or piperacillin, 2 g q8h. If patients are not acutely ill, and must be treated parenterally only because they cannot take medications orally, many clinicians would halve the doses above or lengthen the dosing intervals.

Treatment should be given for 7–14 days. If a parenteral regimen is chosen, it should be changed to an oral regimen as soon as the culture report is available and the patient can tolerate an oral antibiotic. The possibility, however, that a positive urine culture represents asymptomatic bacteriuria or coincidental infection in a patient who actually has an unrecognized respiratory, soft tissue, or another infection must always be kept in mind.

The utility of urine cultures is unclear; they are not cost-effective in ambulatory patients, but are more likely to be useful in the complicated UTIs encountered in long-term care. Follow-up cultures should not be done routinely.

All patients with chronic indwelling urinary catheters become infected. They are more likely to have asymptomatic colonization, asymptomatic infection, complicated antibiotic-resistant infection, and unresponsive infections. Catheters should be removed unless there are no alternatives (very rarely the situation), and intermittent catheterization or absorbent briefs should be used if patients cannot control voiding. Because of the risk of serious and recurrent UTI, catheters should never be used for nursing home staff convenience. Bacteria that cause UTI in catheterized patients are likely to be resistant to TMP/ SMX and febrile infection should usually be empirically treated with a quinolone, such as ofloxacin. The ideal duration of therapy is not known since eradication of bacteriuria is an inappropriate goal—colonization or infection will recur in 100% of patients within a few weeks. At least 2 weeks of therapy, however, is prudent.

Respiratory Infections

Unfortunately, sputum is difficult to obtain and to culture promptly in long-term care patients, with the result that attempts to culture sputum usually yields no growth or an inadequate specimen (10, 20, 28). Therapy must, therefore, be started with the expectation that reliable culture results will not be available to guide treatment decisions. Quinolones are one good initial choice for empiric therapy of respiratory infections, because of their unusually broad range of activity against respiratory pathogens (29). Concerns about limited efficacy in pneumococcal infections remain controversial, but sensitivity data notwithstanding, evidence is accumulating that quinolones differ in their activity against *Streptococcus pneumoniae* and that ofloxacin is clinically effective in pneumococcal respiratory infections (22, 30). In nursing home settings, moreover, Gram-negative bacilli, such as *Haemophilus influenzae, Staphylococcus aureus, Moraxella catarrhalis,* and mixed infection are more common, and pneumococci are encountered relatively infrequently in comparison with their frequency in community-acquired respiratory infections. Quinolones are also active against *Legionella pneumophila,* a serious cause of pneumonia in the elderly patient with chronic lung disease. *Chlamydia pneumoniae* (formerly TWAR strain) may be an important pathogen in multifactorial respiratory infections and, like *C. trachomatis,* is sensitive to ofloxacin and the tetracyclines.

TMP/SMX is also a good empiric antibiotic choice for complicated respiratory infections, although it does not have as favorable tissue penetration or pharmacokinetics as quinolones; it is, however, less expensive. Among the β-lactam antibiotics, amoxicillin/clavulanate and, possibly, cefixime have a sufficiently broad spectrum of activity for empiric use.

If IM parenteral therapy is required, a third-generation cephalosporin such as ceftriaxone, 1 g qday, ceftazidime, or cefoperazone, 1 g q12h are reasonable options. In the acutely ill patient, some clinicians use a 2-g IM/IV loading dose. If IV therapy is necessary, ofloxacin or extended-spectrum penicillins may also be used.

Soft Tissue Infections

In contrast to urinary and respiratory infections, there are few data on which to base empiric therapy for soft tissue infections. If there is underlying vascular insufficiency, or if pressure sores are not properly treated, any antimicrobial regimen, no matter how carefully designed, may fail. Limited-spectrum cephalosporins or dicloxacillin lack activity against Gram-negative bacilli and limited-spectrum penicillins such as amoxicillin lack activity against staphylococci. Amoxicillin/clavulanate, however, has an appropriate spectrum of activity; TMP/SMX is not usually prescribed for soft tissue infections, but its spectrum of activity includes the major pathogens and may be a reasonable choice as well. Quinolones, despite concerns about limited anaerobic activity, have been surprisingly effective in complicated soft tissue infections; their efficacy in the treatment of osteomyelitis may be an important reason for their success (4, 5, 21, 31)

If IM parenteral therapy is chosen, any cephalosporin, such as those listed in Table 3.4, including cefazolin, 1 g q12h, is reasonable initial therapy. Culture of wounds or ulcers is unreliable and is more likely to misguide than to guide therapy. Rather, it is more rational to begin with a broad-spectrum antibiotic empirically, or to broaden therapy if there is a disappointing response to initial narrow-spectrum therapy than to assume that cultures can inform therapeutic decisions. Broad-spectrum IV penicillins that have antistaphylococcal activity such as ampicillin/sulbactam or ticarcillin/clavulanate and IV quinolones (21) are also reasonable choices for empiric therapy. Duration of treatment and the decision to change to oral antimicrobials depend entirely on response to therapy and on the physician's judgment.

Debridement and wound care are equally or more important than antimicrobial therapy in the type of soft tissue infection that occurs in long-term care. Antibiotics, therefore, must not distract clinicians from the more useful surgical and nursing treatment of pressure or ischemic ulcers.

Abdominal Infections

Anaerobic coverage is essential for empiric therapy of abdominal infections. As a single oral agent, only amoxicillin/clavulanate (or chloramphenicol, a still-effective but rarely used drug) has both Gram-negative bacillary and anaerobic coverage. The combination of twice-daily metronidazole and a quinolone gives broader coverage for patients who cannot tolerate amoxicillin/clavulanate or who are allergic to penicillin.

Parenteral therapy has traditionally been cefotetan or cefoxitin, although there is no convincing difference in clinical results when empiric regimens with the second- or third-generation cephalosporins, or the third-generation penicillins have been compared. Most intra-abdominal infections that require parenteral antimicrobial therapy in this group of patients also require surgery or, at least, radiological evaluation for cancer, abscess or fistulae, infarcted or perforated bowel, or gallbladder infection—unless the patient or the family has indicated a wish for nonsurgical therapy only.

References

1. Brumfitt W, Hamilton-Miller J. Methicillin-resistant *Staphylococcus aureus*. N Engl J Med 1989;320:1188.
2. Forstall GJ, Knapp CC, Washington JA. Activity of new quinolones against ciprofloxacin-resistant staphylococci. Antimicrob Agents Chemother 1991;35:1679.
3. Farber BF, et al. A prospective study of nosocomial infections in a chronic care facility. J Am Geriatr Soc 1984;32:499.
4. Yoshikawa TT. Approach to the diagnosis and treatment of the infected older adult. In Hazzard WR, et al. Principles of geriatric medicine and gerontology, 2d ed. 1990:1055.
5. Irvine PW, Van Buren N, Crossley K. Causes for hospitalization of nursing residents: the role of infection. J Am Geriatr Soc 1984;32:103.
6. McCue JD. Gram-negative bacillary bacteremia in the elderly: incidence, ecology, etiology and mortality. J Am Geriatr Soc 1987:35;40.
7. Norman DC, et al. Infections in the nursing home. J Am Geriatr Soc 1987;35:796.
8. Alvarez S, et al. Nosocomial infections in long-term facilities. J Gerontol 1988;43:179.
9. Setia U, Serventi I, Lorenz P. Bacteremia in a long-term care facility. Spectrum and mortality. Arch Intern Med 1984;144:1633.
10. Nunley D, Verghese A, Berk SL. Pneumonia in the nursing-home patient. In: Verghese A, Berk SL, eds. Infections in nursing homes and long-term care facilities 1990:95.
11. Tzias V, Dontas AS, Petrikkos G, et al. Three-day antibiotic therapy in bacteriuria of old age. J Antimicrob Chemother 1990;26:705.
12. Norman DC, et al. Fever and aging. J Am Geriatr Soc 1985;33:859.
13. Gleckman R, Hibert D. Afebrile bacteremia: a phenomenon in geriatric patients. JAMA 1981;243:1478.
14. Finklestein MS, et al. Pneumococcal bacteremia in adults. Age-dependent differences in presentation and in outcome. J Am Geriatr Soc 1983;31:19.
15. Marrie TJ, et al. Community-acquired pneumonia requiring hospitalization. Is it different in the elderly? J Am Geriatr Soc 1985;38:671.
16. Garibaldi RA, Brodine S, Matsumiya S. Infections among patients in nursing homes. N Engl J Med 1981;305:731.

17. Norman DC, Yoshikawa TT. Clinical features of infection and the significance of fever in the elderly nursing-home patient. In Verghese A, Berk SL, eds. Infections in nursing homes and long-term care facilities. 1990:30.

18. Castel SC, Norman DC, Yeh M, et al. Fever response in elderly nursing home residents: are the older truly colder? J Am Geriatr Soc 1991;39:853.

19. Keating H, Klimek J, Levine D, et al. Effect of aging on the clinical significance of fever in ambulatory adult patients. J Am Geriatr Soc 1984;32:282.

20. Harper C, Newton P. Clinical aspects of pneumonia in the elderly veteran. J Am Geriatr Soc 1989;37:867.

21. Lentino JR, Augustinsky JB, Weber TM, Pachucki CT. Therapy of serious skin and soft tissue infection with ofloxacin administered by intravenous and oral route. Chemother 1991;37:70.

22. Gentry LO, Rodriguez-Gomez G, Kohler RB, et al. Parenteral followed by oral ofloxacin for nosocomial pneumonia and community-acquired pneumonia requiring hospitalization. Am Rev Respir Dis 1992;145:31.

23. Nicolle LE, Bjornson J, Harding GKM, et al. Bacteriuria in elderly institutionalized men. N Engl J Med 1983;309:1420.

24. Boscia JA, Abrutyn E, Kaye D. Asymptomatic bacteriuria in elderly persons: treat or do not treat? Ann Intern Med 1987;106:764.

25. Zhanel GG, Godfrey KM, Harding MD, Guay DR. Asymptomatic bacteriuria. Which patients should be treated? Arch Intern Med 1990;150:1389.

26. Wise R. The pharmacokinetics of the oral cephalosporins—a review. J Antimicrob Chemother 1990;26(Suppl E):13.

27. Israel D, Polk RE. Focus on clarithromycin and azithromycin: two new macrolide antibiotics. Hosp Form 1992;27:115.

28. Verghese A, Berk SL. Bacterial pneumonia in the elderly. Clin Rpt Aging 1989;3:1.

29. Peterson PK, Stein D. Guay DR, et al. Prospective study of lower respiratory tract infections in an extended care nursing home program: potential role of oral ciprofloxacin. Am J Med 1988;85:164.

30. Sanders WE, Morris JF, Alessi P, et al. Oral ofloxacin for the treatment of acute bacterial pneumonia: use of a nontraditional protocol to compare experimental therapy with "usual care" in a multicenter clinical trial. Am J Med 1991;91:261.

31. Rubenstein E, Adam D, Moellering R, Waldvogel F, eds. International symposium on new quinolones. Rev Infect Dis 1989;11(Suppl 5):1.

4

Treatment of Depression and Depressive Symptoms

Jack D. McCue

There have been few studies to guide physicians in the diagnosis and management of depression in elderly patients who live in long-term care settings; nearly all studies have focused on community-dwelling or acutely hospitalized elderly patients. The few studies that have examined the relative frequency of depressive symptoms, chronic illnesses with symptoms of depression, and clinical depression in elderly long-term care residents have reported, however, a much higher prevalence of clinical depression, depressive symptoms, and depressive symptoms associated with dementia than has been reported in community-dwelling elders (1–4). Overall, at least one-third of patients in long-term care have either clinical depression or depressive symptoms, in comparison with community-dwelling elderly who have a prevalence of major depression of 1–3% and a prevalence of depressive symptoms of about 15% (5, 6).

Although it is known that elderly depressed patients experience a high mortality—Rovner et al. (4) reported a 31% 1-year survival for long-term care patients with major depression—data on the benefits and perils of drug or electroconvulsive therapy in this medically complicated and fragile population are inconclusive and conflicting (4–6). Although many patients respond to treatment with a gratifying resolution of symptoms, many do not; relapses on therapy or after discontinuation of antidepressants are common, and drug intolerance that prevents administration of full therapeutic doses of antidepressants is very common.

DIAGNOSIS OF DEPRESSION IN LONG-TERM CARE

Clinicians typically establish the diagnosis of depression in the elderly in three ways: formal psychiatric evaluation, use of screening instruments that have been validated for the elderly, and clinical suspicion plus a response to antidepressant.

43

Table 4.1.   Diagnostic Criteria for Clinical Depression of Late Life[a]

Major criteria
  Either depressed mood and/or loss of interest or pleasure
Minor criteria
  Three or four of the following (for a total of five)
    Weight change
    Sleep disturbance
    Psychomotor agitation or retardation
    Fatigue
    Feelings of worthlessness
    Difficulty concentrating
    Recurrent thoughts of death

[a]Adapted, in part, from Blazer DG. Depression. In: Hazzard WR, Andres R, Bierman EL, Blass JP, eds. Principles of geriatric medicine and gerontology, 2nd ed. New York: McGraw-Hill, 1990:1010.

Formal Psychiatric Assessment

The definitive diagnosis of clinical or major depression is usually based on the DSM-IIIR criteria, summarized in Table 4.1. The diagnosis requires the presence of one or two of the major criteria, plus three or four of the minor criteria, for a total of five signs or symptoms. The advantage of using DSM-IIIR standards for diagnosing depression lies primarily in the consistency with which these criteria have been applied in geropsychiatric research. It is clear, however, that many patients who would benefit from treatment for depression do not meet strict diagnostic criteria for clinical depression; in other words, the criteria, while reliably specific in most populations, may not be sensitive enough to satisfy the needs of clinicians working with medically complicated older patients. More problematic, the communication skills required to respond to the diagnostic questioning required for DSM-IIIR criteria may be lacking in long-term care patients with dementia, stroke, or other neurological disorders.

Of equal concern for the chronically ill long-term care patient, the minor criteria are too nonspecific. Any may be encountered in the physically ill or frail elderly who do not otherwise appear to be depressed or who do not respond to treatment with antidepressant medication.

Screening Instruments

A variety of self-administered and doctor- or nurse-administered screening instruments for depression have been validated for the community-dwelling elderly (7). The utility of these instruments for long-term care patients is less certain; these instruments, which are designed to be sensitive to avoid missing atypical or subtle presentations of depression, may be too time-consuming and give too many false-positive results to be useful in long-term care patients in whom depressive symptoms are common. They are, nevertheless, an important basic tool for the evaluation of functionally impaired older persons.

Clinical Suspicion and Response to Empiric Therapy

Long-term care patients (or family and guardians, in some cases) who can communicate effectively may be able to help establish the diagnosis of depression for the inquiring clinician by their responses to a few straightforward screening questions, such as those suggested by Kane et al. (8) (Table 4.2) In most cases, however, the diagnosis of significant

---

Table 4.2. A "Clinical Suspicion" Depression Screen[a]

For each of the following questions, which description comes closest to the way you have been feeling during the past month?

a. How much of the time, during the past month, has your health limited your social activities (like visiting friends or relatives)?
b. How much of the time, during the past month, have you been a very nervous person?
c. During the past month, how much of the time have you felt calm and peaceful?
d. How much of the time, during the past month, have you felt downhearted and blue?
e. During the past month, how much of the time have you been a happy person?
f. How often, during the past month, have you felt so down in the dumps that nothing could cheer you up?
g. During the past month, how often has feeling depressed interfered with what you usually do?
h. During the past month, how often did you feel that you had nothing to look forward to?
i. How often have you felt like crying during the past month?
j. During the past month, how often did you feel like life isn't worth living anymore?

---

[a]Adapted, in part, from Kane RL, Ouslander JG, Abrass IB. Essentials of clinical geriatrics, 2nd ed. New York: McGraw-Hill, 1989.

depressive symptoms or clinical depression ultimately rests on the symptomatic response to empiric antidepressant therapy. A new sleep disturbance, unexplained weight loss, refusal to participate in social activities or rehabilitation, refusal to take medication, or "taking to bed" are examples of nonspecific symptoms that may respond to antidepressant therapy, regardless of whether it is possible to make a formal diagnosis of clinical depression.

Predicting Response to Therapy

There are no reliable physiological or clinical predictors of which patients will respond to empiric drug therapy (9) (Table 4.3). Earlier studies suggesting that a stable personality before the onset of depression, a moderate severity of depression, the absence of preceding psychiatric or physical illness, and the absence of dementia, which have been cited in the past as diagnostic indicators of responsiveness to tricyclic antidepressants, are less reliable than once thought.

PRACTICAL DIAGNOSTIC CATEGORIES

Listed in Table 4.4 are some psychiatric and nonpsychiatric diagnoses that, in addition to clinical depression, may be responsible for depressive symptoms in late life. Some, such as those listed under mood disorders,

Table 4.3.   Symptoms Suggestive of Responsive Depression of Late Life[a]

Loss of interest or pleasure
Lack of response to pleasure stimuli
Symptoms worse each morning
Significant weight loss
Previous response to antidepressants
Previous depression with remission
Psychotic symptoms
Lack of rapid mood cycling
Absence of dementia
Retarded depression rather than agitated depression (mixed depression/anxiety)
Pure major depression versus double depression (major depression plus dysthymia)

[a]Adapted, in part, from Blazer DG. Depression. In: Hazzard WR, Andres R, Bierman EL, Blass JP, eds. Principles of geriatric medicine and gerontology, 2nd ed. New York: McGraw-Hill, 1990:1010; neither validated nor necessarily reliable for the type of depression encountered in long-term care.

Table 4.4.   Differential Diagnosis of Depressive Symptoms in Late Life

Mood Disorders
  Clinical depression
  Dysthymia (depressive neurosis)
  Bipolar disorder, depressed
Adjustment disorders
  Depressive reaction to losses
  Bereavement
Organic causes
  Dementia with associated depression
  Physical illness (e.g., hypothyroidism, stroke, carcinoma of the pancreas)
Medications, such as
  Psychotropics, especially benzodiazepines
  Cardiovasculars, especially β-blockers, reserpine, methyldopa
  Antiseizure medications
Others
  Extreme old age with dementia
  Pseudodepression (chronic disease causing depressive symptoms)
  Dying ("taking to bed")
  "Institutionitis"

are DSM-IIIR diagnoses; some diagnoses, such as the ill-defined disorders listed under "others" describe circumstances in which often severe depressive symptoms occur, particularly in the long-term care setting. Only the mood disorders typically respond completely to antidepressant pharmacotherapy, although some of the symptoms associated with the others may improve with drug treatment. The challenge for clinicians, more than making a precise diagnosis, is determining who, of their long-term care patients, may improve with therapy, who will experience adverse effects of drug treatment without benefit, and who will require an aggressive, persistent approach to treatment.

Extreme age is associated with anorexia and weight loss in some patients, for which no explanation can be found other than, possibly, the results of brain aging (10–12). "Taking to bed" or "giving up" is a syndrome of rapid functional decline and apathy in which only about one-half of patients have clearly identifiable precipitating medical events (13). A variety of diseases such as hypothyroidism, stroke, and malignancy may cause depressive symptoms (14, 15). Pseudodepression is the name given to the constellation of nonspecific depressive symptoms caused by or associated with multiple chronic illnesses and disabilities (16).

The clinical evaluation of possibly depressed patients is no different from the careful, pragmatic evaluation that all elderly patients with functional disabilities or chronic illness should receive. This type of evaluation, which relies more on history, physical, and interdisciplinary assessment than on laboratory testing, is summarized in the major geriatric texts (8, 17, 18).

PRAGMATIC APPROACH TO THERAPY

Summarized in Table 4.5 are characteristics of selected antidepressant drugs that are useful in long-term care settings. Before starting antidepressant drug therapy, however, the first step in treatment is to stop *all* drugs that are not essential: not only may these medications be the *cause* of the depressive symptoms, many will complicate therapy by causing drug interactions. Particular attention must be paid to all psychotropics, such as sedatives, sleeping medications, antipsychotics, and anxiolytics. Anticonvulsants such as phenytoin are a frequently unrecognized cause of depressive symptoms, as are cardiovascular agents such as propranolol and central-blocker antihypertensives. Relatively less fat-soluble β-blockers, such as atenolol, may be less likely to cause depression (19).

Tricyclics

Tricyclic antidepressants (and heterocyclic drugs, such as trazodone) have similar side-effect profiles, although the intensity of adverse symptoms varies with the agent chosen. Although nortriptyline has been studied more extensively in the elderly (5), desipramine causes less sedation and is, thus, the tricyclic agent that is usually chosen first. Typically, it is begun at a low initial dose of 25 mg at bedtime. Depending on the severity of depressive symptoms and comorbid brain

---

. . . desipramine causes less sedation and is, thus, the tricyclic agent that is usually chosen first.

Table 4.5.   Antidepressant Therapy for the Frail Elderly[a]

Antidepressant and Chemical Category	Frail Elderly Doses[b] (Initial/Maintenance)	Relative Sedation	Relative Anticholinergic Effect	Relative Postural Hypotension
Heterocyclics				
Desipramine (generic)	10 mg/100 mg qhs	+	+	++
Nortriptyline (Pamelor)	10 mg/100 mg qhs	++	+	+
Doxepin (generic)	10 mg/100 mg qhs	+++	+++	+++
Others				
Trazodone (generic)	50 mg/200 mg qhs	+++	0	++
Fluoxetine (Prozac)	10 mg/20 mg qday	0	0	0
Sertraline (Zoloff)	25 mg/100 mg qday	+	+	0
Phenelzine (Nardil)	15 mg/45 mg qday	+	0	+++
Bupropion (Wellbutrin)	50 mg/100 mg qday	0	0	0
Alprazolam (Xanax)	0.25 mg/0.5 mg b.i.d.	+++	0	0

[a]From Potter WZ, Rudorfer MV, Manji H. The pharmacologic treatment of depression. N Engl J Med 1991;325:633; and Blazer D. Depression in the elderly. N Engl J Med 1989;320:164.
[b]Higher doses may need to be split into b.i.d. or t.i.d. dosing to minimize side effects.

disease (which increases the risk of delirium or somnolence), the dose is increased by 25–50 mg every 3–7 days. The usual maintenance dose is 75–100 mg; rarely is 150 mg required, and only a few elderly patients will tolerate doses higher than 150 mg without severe adverse effects.

When patients begin to respond, the same dose should be maintained; improvement usually continues at that dose and higher doses do not yield greater benefits. A divided dose during daytime rather than a single bedtime dose may reduce morning postural hypotension, but at the cost of increased sedation and dry mouth. There is little role for serum levels of tricyclics in the elderly, except to document that a severely depressed but nonresponsive patient who is receiving 150 mg or more has reasonable or "therapeutic" serum concentrations.

If patients do not respond to 75–100 mg of desipramine, it is unlikely that they will respond to other heterocyclics, although it is reasonable to try fluoxetine or sertralene because of their low side-effect profiles. As little as 10 mg of fluoxetine daily or every other day is a reasonable initial dose, and doses of above 20 mg cause delirium more commonly than desipramine; the weight loss that is associated with higher doses of fluoxetine may also present a special problem in the elderly. There is less experience in the elderly with sertraline—reasonable initial dose is 50 mg at supper or breakfast, with slow titration up to a daily dose of 150 mg (20).

Low doses of tricyclic antidepressants (25–50 mg at bedtime) or alprazolam (0.25–0.5 mg twice daily) may be helpful in the atypical depressive syndromes. Reduction of anxiety, raising of pain threshold, improved sleep, and perhaps improved appetite (a common and troublesome side effect of the tricyclic agents in younger patients) may make the chronically ill long-term care patient with depressive symptoms more comfortable.

Other Antidepressants

The monoamine oxidase inhibitor antidepressant L-deprenyl has received attention recently for its utility in retarding the onset of symptoms of Parkinson's disease, but tends to be rarely used for depression in the elderly. The dietary restrictions that make physicians reluctant to use this class of drugs (some cheeses, canned fish and meat, red wines, chocolate), however, are unnecessary for lower dose regimens; if required, they are easier to implement in long-term care where there is greater control over diet. Patients who do not respond to heterocyclics but appear to have a clinical depression may respond well to monoamine oxidase (MAO) inhibitors, but those who do not tolerate tricyclic agents will probably not tolerate phenelzine or tranylcypromine either.

Bupropion, which is chemically unrelated to the heterocyclic agents, has a promising side-effect profile, but has not been studied as extensively as the other antidepressants in the elderly, and its efficacy in the treatment of depression is not yet clear (9).

Alprazolam, a benzodiazepine, is an effective antidepressant in high doses (3 mg per day) in younger patients, but older patients do not tolerate the sedation that often occurs with higher doses. Because of its favorable side-effect profile, however, low doses may be helpful for atypical depressions, especially those associated with anxiety or agitation, such as pseudodepression or taking to bed.

Stimulants, such as methylphenidate or triiodothyronine, may be tried for resistant cases, but rarely work and never give lasting remissions. Electroconvulsive therapy may be helpful in resistant cases and is an underutilized treatment for clinical depression in general. Agitated patients, especially those who appear to be cycling between apathy and agitation, may benefit from lithium even though the diagnosis of bipolar disorder is not clearly apparent.

References

1. Hyer L, Blazer DG. Depression in long-term care facilities. In: Blazer DG, ed. Depression in late life. St. Louis: CV Mosby, 1982.
2. Rovner BW, Kafonek S, Filipp L, et al. Prevalence of mental illness in a community nursing home. Am J Psychiatry 1986;143:1446.
3. Teeter RB, et al. Psychiatric disturbances of aged patients in skilled nursing homes. Am J Psychiatry 1976;133:1430.
4. Rovner BW, German PS, Brant LJ, et al. Depression and mortality in nursing homes. JAMA 1991;265:993.
5. Katz IR, Curlik S, Lesher EL. Use of antidepressants in the frail elderly. When, why, and how. Clin Geriatr Med 1988;4:203.
6. Blazer DG. Depression. In: Hazzard WR, Andres R, Bierman EL, Blass JP, eds. Principles of geriatric medicine and gerontology, 2nd ed. New York: McGraw-Hill, 1990:1010.

7. Kane RL, Kane RA. Assessing the elderly: a practical guide to measurement. Lexington, MA: Heath, 1981.
8. Kane RL, Ouslander JG, Abrass IB. Essentials of clinical geriatrics, 2nd ed. New York: McGraw-Hill, 1989.
9. Potter WZ, Rudorfer MV, Manji H. The pharmacologic treatment of depression. N Engl J Med 1991;325:633.
10. Thompson MP, Morris LK. Unexplained weight loss in the ambulatory elderly. J Am Geriatr Soc 1991;39:497.
11. Morley JE, Silver AJ. Anorexia in the elderly. Neurobiol Aging 1988;9:9.
12. Jarvik LF. Aging of the brain: how can we prevent it? Gerontologist 1988;26:739.
13. Clark LP, Dion DM, Barker WH. Taking to bed. J Am Geriatr Soc 1990;38:967.
14. Graham H, Livesley B. Dying as a diagnosis: difficulties of communication and management in elderly patients. Lancet 1983;2:670.
15. Streim JE, Marshall JR. The dying elderly patient. Am Fam Physician 1988;38:175.
16. Coulehan JL, Schulberg HC, Block MR, et al. Medical comorbidity of major depressive disorder in a primary medical practice. Arch Intern Med 1990;150:2363.
17. Hazzard WR, Andres R, Bierman EL, Blass JP, eds. Principles of geriatric medicine and gerontology, 2nd ed. New York: McGraw-Hill, 1990.
18. Cassel CK, Riesenberg DE, Sorensen LB, Walsh JR, eds. Geriatric medicine, 2nd ed. New York: Springer-Verlag, 1990.
19. Wallin JD, Shah SV. β-Adrenergic blocking agents in the treatment of hypertension. Arch Intern Med 1987;147:654.
20. Guthrie SK. Setraline: a new serotonin reuptake blocker. DICP Ann Pharmacother 1991;25:952.
21. Blazer D. Depression in the elderly. N Engl J Med 1989;320:164.

5

Antihypertensive Therapy

Jack D. McCue

The treatment of mild-to-moderate hypertension for most asymptomatic elderly patients who reside in long-term care facilities may not be beneficial, either in terms of improvement in the quality or of extension of the quantity of life. There are, moreover, some indications that at greatly advanced age the risks of high blood pressure treatment exceed the benefits, resulting in an increase in mortality and morbidity (1–3). Therapy should not be initiated, therefore, until the goals of treatment, such as improving symptoms of ischemic heart disease or congestive heart failure (CHF), are clearly articulated.

If, however, prevention of future occlusive vascular events such as stroke or myocardial infarction is the treatment goal, a realistic assessment of the actual risk of an ischemic event is important. Such an assessment must take into account a realistic estimation of the patient's life expectancy (most patients in long-term care live fewer than 3 years after permanent "placement") and the presence of other risk factors for atherosclerotic vascular disease before exposing a very elderly patient to the potential hazard of morbidity or diminished quality of life resulting from adverse effects of antihypertensive therapy during his or her few remaining years of life.

DECISION TO TREAT

There is no convincing scientific support for the treatment of asymptomatic hypertension of chronically ill or disabled patients who are over 80 years of age and reside in long-term care facilities. Definitive studies have been performed only in populations of relatively healthy elderly patients who are capable of independent living and in whom serious chronic diseases, such as ischemic heart disease or neurological disorders, or mild renal insufficiency have been excluded (1–10). Most elderly patients living in long-term care have multiple chronic diseases that limit life expectancy and complicate drug therapy. In addition, unlike independently living elderly hypertensives, long-term care patients have other risk factors such as diet, exercise, or smoking either controlled or under medical supervision. In summary, treatment of "biologically young" hypertensives under the age of 80 years has been proved beneficial, and treatment of relatively healthy patients past the age of 80 is reasonable, despite lack of supporting data that therapy is beneficial. Treatment of the frail very elderly hypertensive, however, should be undertaken primarily for symptomatic conditions and should employ medications with a low profile of adverse effects.

The large-scale studies of the benefits of treatment of hypertension in the elderly that were performed in the last decade and were summarized by Applegate and others (2, 3, 11) have led to several important conclusions that may influence the decision to treat mild-to-moderate hypertension in the elderly patient residing in a long-term care facility:

1. The incidence of "vascular events" such as new ischemic cardiovascular or neurovascular symptoms or infarctions is reduced by about 30% in relatively healthy patients under 80 years old, but possibly not for older patients. The absolute benefit for the younger elderly, however, is far less impressive; independently living older patients experienced a reduction of less than 1% in their absolute risk of a new vascular event from the baseline incidence of 2–3% of new vascular events per year (e.g., new onset of angina pectoris, transient ischemic attacks, stroke, or myocardial infarction).

2. None of the major studies has shown a significant reduction in overall mortality with treatment of mild-to-moderate hypertension of patients over 65 years old, including the recently reported SHEP study (systolic hypertension in the elderly project) (4). Some data, in fact, indicate that overall mortality may actually increase with treatment of hypertension in some patients over the age of 80 years (2).

   The type of patient residing in long-term care facilities may be at special risk for harm resulting from aggressive lowering of diastolic blood pressure, resulting in the so-called "J-curve phenomenon" in which the beneficial effect on morbidity and mortality of treatment (the downward slope of the letter J) levels off and becomes detrimental (the curve and rising tail of the letter J) with increasing age (11). The explanation for the J-curve phenomenon is unclear, although it is hypothesized that the hypertrophied or fibrotic left ventricle typical of hypertensive and atherosclerotic heart disease in the very elderly patient is unable to sustain diastolic blood pressure at the level required for coronary and cerebral blood flow when hypertension is treated aggressively.

Other hypotheses have been advanced to explain the apparent loss of benefit of treatment of hypertension after the age of 80 years: The abbreviated absolute life expectancy, especially of the old-old patients makes small improvements undetectable; electrolyte abnormalities induced by diuretics or angiotensin-converting enzyme (ACE), inhibitors superimposed on underlying coronary disease may induce lethal arrhythmias; reduced cerebral or renal perfusion as a result of reduced arterial pressure cause comorbid complications that shorten survival; adverse drug reactions such as confusion or postural hypotension from β-blockers or central blockers, such as propranolol or clonidine, lead to acute illnesses, injuries, or hosptialization.

3. While most studies of the benefits of antihypertensive therapy have concentrated on diastolic hypertension, there appears to be little difference in the risks of nontreatment or benefits of treatment between systolic-diastolic and isolated systolic hypertension.

4. Although it is universally observed that systolic blood pressure tends to rise with age, systolic hypertension is a disease process and not a normal manifestation of aging. Unlike systolic pressure, diastolic blood pressure does not rise with increasing age in previously normotensive elderly persons (12).

CONSIDERATIONS IN THE DECISION TO TREAT THE ELDERLY HYPERTENSIVE

Age

Independently living, relatively healthy patients aged 65–80 years old should generally be treated by the same criteria as younger patients. Most of these patients have a life expectancy of 10–30 years and may benefit from the treatment of mild hypertension. Patients older than 80 years (even if healthy) and younger elders with serious chronic diseases or functional disabilities requiring residence in a long-term care facility will probably not benefit from treatment of mild-to-moderate hypertension either in terms of greater life expectancy or better quality of life

(Table 5.1). Whether gender should be part of the decision to treat is not known, but some data indicate that treatment of mild-to-moderate hypertension in white women may have no benefit or may even increase risk of mortality and vascular events (13).

Mild Hypertension and Adverse Drug Reactions (ADRs)

Therapy for elderly long-term care patients with blood pressures below 160/100 mm Hg, regardless of age, should be instituted only after careful consideration of the potential risks and benefits. Moreover, therapy should not be continued in the face of adverse events that lead to a deterioration in the quality of life. Hence, the development of postural hypotension, sleep disturbances, or confusion should lead to discontinuation of therapy, unless treatment is specifically directed at symptoms that require short-term treatment. While relatively healthy, independently living elders do not seem to experience a higher incidence of adverse events with antihypertensive therapy than younger patients,

Table 5.1.   Recommendations for Treatment of Elevated Blood Pressure in the Elderly Residing in Long-term Care[a]

Drug therapy for
  Systolic and diastolic hypertension with diastolic > 100 mm Hg
  Isolated systolic hypertension > 180 mm Hg
Try to avoid drug therapy or use nondrug therapy if possible
  Systolic and diastolic hypertension with systolic 160–180 mm Hg and diastolic 95–100 mm Hg
  Isolated systolic hypertension 160–180 mm Hg, especially with diastolic pressures < 80 mm Hg
No therapy unless symptoms or specific indications are present
  Systolic hypertension 140–160 mm Hg
  Diastolic hypertension 90–95 mm Hg
  Drug side-effects that impair quality of life are likely
No therapy if
  Significant quality-of-life deterioration occurs with therapy
  Brief life expectancy or very poor quality of life are present
  Severe dementia or chronic vegetative state are present

[a]Adapted, in part, from Applegate WB. High blood pressure treatment in the elderly. Clin Geriatr Med 1992;8:103.

this is unlikely to be the case with the fragile, chronically ill patients in long-term care facilities.

End-organ Damage

The presence of end-organ damage may have a special meaning in the elderly, in that it may predict imminent risk of cardiovascular, renovascular, or neurovascular complications. Hence, a patient with left ventricular hypertrophy (LVH), hypertensive renal disease, or past stroke probably has advanced clinical hypertensive disease, and may benefit more from treatment of hypertension than patients without clinically detectable end-organ damage. On the other hand, end-organ damage may also increase the risks of antihypertensive therapy, resulting in decreased cardiac output, renal insufficiency, diminished cognition, or postural hypotension. There is growing, convincing evidence that the presence of LVH imposes an independent risk for mortality and morbidity in older hypertensive patients (15–18).

Pseudohypertension

A relatively uncommon condition found in an occasional elderly patient with rigid or calcified brachial arteries, pseudohypertension is the artifactual overestimation of intra-arterial blood pressure by the standard indirect blood pressure measurement using an arm cuff. The Osler Maneuver, in which the brachial and radial arteries are found to be still palpable after the cuff pressure has been inflated above the systolic pressure, can be used to screen for possible pseudohypertension (12).

A more common reason for a blood pressure reading that is misleading is so-called white-coat hypertension—a form of labile hypertension in which blood pressures tend to rise significantly only when the pressure is being taken. Such patients usually are otherwise normotensive and are at little if any increased risk for complications from hypertension. White-coat hypertension is present in up to 20% of younger patients, and probably complicates the management of at least an equal number of elderly patients (18).

EVALUATION OF HYPERTENSION IN LONG-TERM CARE

Laboratory evaluation of hypertension beyond the routine testing of renal function, electrolytes, chest x-ray, and electrocardiogram should be prompted by poor response to conservative blood pressure management and patient willingness to accept definitive treatment. Hence, one should not search for renal artery stenosis or hyperaldosteronism unless invasive, definitive management can be justified by the patient's general condition, life-expectancy, and willingness to accept hospitalization and the complications of invasive therapy. The most common cause of secondary hypertension or worsening of stable familial hypertension in the elderly is renal artery stenosis, of which some cases are identifiable by careful search for flank or abdominal bruits. Other causes of secondary hypertension are rare and definitive treatment is rarely justifiable in the elderly nursing home patient; a search for secondary causes is never justifiable in patients who are well controlled on antihypertensive therapy.

THERAPY

Patients under age 65–80 years who are relatively healthy may benefit from the treatment of asymptomatic mild-to-moderate hypertension. Patients over 80 years, even if in good health, and younger elderly patients with chronic diseases who reside in long-term care may not benefit from antihypertensive therapy. There is some evidence that the very elderly may experience an increase in mortality from the complications of therapy itself, or from aggressive treatment of isolated systolic hypertension that results in excessive lowering of diastolic blood pressure. Although future studies may facilitate prospective identification of patients at special risk of complications from lowering of diastolic blood pressure, at present, prudence dictates either very gentle treatment or nontreatment of patients with systolic hypertension whose diastolic blood pressure is below 80 mm Hg. When mild diastolic hypertension is encountered, there should be reluctance to treat to lower diastolic pressures to between 95 and 100 mm Hg because of probable lack of benefit, and diastolic blood pressure

Patients over 80 years, even if in good health, and younger elderly patients with chronic diseases who reside in long-term care may not benefit from antihypertensive therapy.

elevations between 90 and 95 mm Hg should not be treated. In addition, care should be taken not to reduce systolic blood pressure below 135–140 mm Hg in the elderly (3).

Nonpharmacological treatment, such as sodium restriction and weight loss, may be more feasible for patients who are under close dietary supervision, such as those in long-term care, than for younger, independently living patients, and may have a modest effect on blood pressure control (19). It is possible that exercise would have a similar beneficial effect, but the ability to exercise is limited in most debilitated or frail elderly patients.

Table 5.2 summarizes some of the drugs that might be considered first

Table 5.2. Recommendations for Initial Therapy of Hypertension in the Elderly Residing in Long-term Care Facilities

Drug	Initial Dose	Adverse Effects
Calcium-channel blockers		Constipation
Sustained-release		
Verapamil (Calan-SR or	60–120 mg qday	
Verelan), diltiazem (Cardizem-SR), or nifedipine		
(Procardia-XL)	60–90 mg qday	
Diuretics		
Hydrochlorothiazide or	25 mg qday	Dehydration, azotemia,
hydrochlorothiazide-triamterene		hypokalemia, hyponatremia, arrhythmias, postural hypotension
β-Blockers	25 mg qday	CHF, confusion, worsening of
Atenolol (Lopressor)		chronic obstructive pulmonary disease
α-Blockers		
Terazosin (Hytrin) or	1 mg qday	
doxazosin (Cardura)		
ACE-inhibitors		
Lisinopril (Prinivil, Zestril) or	2.5 mg qday	Hyperkalemia, unpredictable
enalapril (Vasotec)	5 mg qday	renal failure

if therapy is indicated for the treatment of either systolic or combined systolic-diastolic hypertension in the elderly, with emphasis on preference for initial single-drug, single-dose therapy. Because of their adverse effects, diuretics are now considered second-line therapy for frail elderly patients by many geriatricians, despite the extensive data accumulated on the benefit of diuretics in the treatment of relatively healthy, independently living elderly hypertensives (3).

Calcium-Blockers

Theoretically, the best choice for single-agent therapy of the elderly hypertensive is a long-acting calcium-blocker. In comparison to diuretics, central-blockers, and β-blockers, however, there have been relatively few studies of calcium-blockers in the elderly, and no large placebo-controlled trials. Widespread clinical experience indicates that they are well tolerated, tend not to cause postural hypotension, tend to lower systolic blood pressure more than the diastolic pressure, and do not cause confusion or sedation. An additional benefit of calcium channel-blocker therapy is the potential reversibility of LVH and its complications, which does not occur with diuretics or central blockers (20–22). There is a greater choice of verapamil preparations than other calcium channel-blockers, including generic regular verapamil, and several sustained-release forms. The major concerns in frail elderly patients are occasional deterioration in cardiac output, constipation, and a potential for drug interactions with digoxin.

Diuretics

Diuretics are a problematic treatment option. On the positive side, the thiazide diuretics are available in inexpensive generic forms, including the commonly used hydrochlorothiazide-triamterene combination that avoids the complication of hypokalemia. They may be given once daily, and several major, large studies have demonstrated them to be well tolerated and effective in relatively healthy, independently living elderly patients (3, 4, 23). Concerns related to adverse effects on serum lipids are of unknown relevance and probably represent an insignificant concern for the elderly population in long-term care (24).

On the negative side, diuretics are physiologically a poor choice for elderly patients, who are susceptible to dehydration, azotemia, and electrolyte disturbances with secondary arrhythmias due to underlying coronary disease or left ventricular hypertrophy. They may worsen osteoporosis and predispose to postural hypotension, which could cause lethal hip fractures (25). The availability of alternative agents has tended to relegate diuretics, therefore, to second-step therapy when moderate doses of a single agent such as a calcium channel-blocker, α-blocker, or β-blocker are ineffective. Low doses of a thiazide should be used; higher doses may disproportionately increase the risk of toxicity without improving blood pressure control. Nonthiazide diuretics have little role as single-agent therapy, although furosemide, which may be less effective and more toxic than thiazides (25), may be useful as second-step therapy in the setting of mild renal insufficiency.

β-Blockers

As is the case with diuretics, β-blockers are not physiologically ideal therapy for elderly hypertensives. Their central nervous system and cardiopulmonary toxicity, which can lead to depression, cognitive slowing, confusion, worsening of chronic obstructive lung disease, and CHF, are more likely to be problematic for the frail chronically ill elderly. On the other hand, large trials in relatively healthy elderly have shown them to be effective and well tolerated when used with a diuretic (26, 27); they can be used once daily, and newer β-blockers that have not been extensively tested in the elderly, may have a reduced potential for inducing congestive heart failure. Atenolol may incur a lesser risk of depressive symptoms and confusion, and is usually preferred over lipid-soluble agents such as propranolol (28).

ACE-inhibitors

Rarely effective as single agents, ACE-inhibitors may be useful when combined with a diuretic (29)—so much so that one should add the diuretic cautiously in patients with impaired cardiac reserve due to LVH, diabetic vascular disease, or coronary disease. Their predilection to cause renal insufficiency unpredictably and the occasional occurrence of the poorly understood "ACE-inhibitor cough," which may be caused by any of the ACE-inhibitors and may resolve very slowly after drug discontinuation, make them useful in the elderly primarily for difficult-to-treat hypertension, perhaps known high-renin hypertension, or hypertension combined with CHF (30). Patients at risk for CHF because of advanced hypertensive heart disease with LVH may benefit from ACE-inhibitor therapy, which may forestall the development of CHF (31).

α-Blockers

Older agents such as prazosin tend to cause unacceptable postural hypotension in elderly patients, especially at the initiation of therapy. Newer α-blockers, such as doxazosin or terazosin, however, are effective and better tolerated in the elderly. They have the additional advantage of once-daily administration and are priced comparably to the calcium-blockers. They are a reasonable selection for single-agent therapy if calcium-blockers are ineffective or not tolerated.

Central-blockers

Most other antihypertensive agents, such as α-methyl dopa, reserpine, or clonidine, tend to cause unacceptable sedation or confusion, especially in the presence of underlying central nervous system disease. They should be used with reluctance and, when encountered in the chronic regimens of long-term care patients, should be discontinued in favor of other agents with less potential for central nervous system toxicity.

References

1. Amery A, Birkenhager W, Brixko R, et al. Efficacy of antihypertensive drug treatment according to age, sex, blood pressure, and previous cardiovascular disease in patients over the age of 60. Lancet 1986;1:589.
2. Applegate WB. Hypertension in elderly patients. Ann Intern Med 1989;110:901.
3. Applegate WB. High blood pressure treatment in the elderly. Clin Geriatr Med 1992;8:103.
4. SHEP Cooperative Research Group. Prevention of stroke by antihypertensive drug treatment in older persons with isolated systolic hypertension. JAMA 1991;265:3255.
5. Hypertension Detection and Follow-up Program Cooperative Group. Persistence of

reduction in blood pressure and mortality participants in the Hypertension Detection and Follow-up Program. JAMA 1988;259:2113.

6. Hypertension Detection Follow-up Cooperative Group. 5 year findings of the hypertension detection follow-up program. JAMA 1979;242:2562.

7. Management Committee of the Australian National Blood Pressure Study. Prognostic factors in the treatment of mild hypertension. Circulation 1984;69:668.

8. National Heart Foundation of Australia. Treatment of mild hypertension in the elderly. Med J Austral 1981;247:633.

9. Applegate WB, Vander ZR, Dismike SE, et al. Control of systolic blood pressure in elderly black patients. J Am Geriatr Soc 1982;30:391.

10. Hulley SB, Furberg CD, Gurland B, et al. Systolic hypertension in the elderly program: antihypertensive efficacy of chlorthalidone. Am J Cardiol 1985;56:913.

11. Cruickshank JM, Thorp JM, Zacharias FJ. Benefits and potential harm of lowering high blood pressure. Lancet 1987;1:581.

12. Zachariah PK, Sheps SG, Bailey KR, et al. Age related characteristics of ambulatory blood pressure load and mean blood pressure in normotensive subjects. JAMA 1991;265:1414.

13. Anastos K, Charney P, Charon RA, et al. Hypertension in women: what is really known? Ann Intern Med 1991;115:286.

14. Messerli FH, Ventura HO, Elizardi DJ, et al. Hypertension and sudden death: increased ventricular ectopic activity in left ventricular hypertrophy. Am J Med 1984;77:18.

15. Levy D, Anderson KM, Savage DD, et al. Risk of ventricular arrhythmias in left ventricular hypertrophy: The Framingham heart study. Am J Cardiol 1987;60:560.

16. Devereaux RB. Importance of left ventricular mass as a predictor of cardiovascular morbidity in hypertension. Am J Hypertens 1989;2:650.

17. Kannell WB, Levy D, Cupplles LA. Left ventricular hypertrophy and risk of cardiac failure: Insights from the Framingham study. J Cardiovasc Pharmacol 1987;10(Suppl 6):S135.

18. Pickering TG, James GD, Boddie C, et al. How common is white coat hypertension? JAMA 1988;259:225.

19. Mader SL, Josephson KR, Rubenstein LZ. Low prevalence of postural hypotension among community dwelling elderly. JAMA 1987;258:1511.

20. Grandi AM, Venco A, Bertolini A, et al. Left ventricular function after reversal of myocardial hypertrophy in systemic hypertension, and response to acute increase of afterload by cold pressor test. Am J Cardiol 1992;69:1439.

21. Messerli FH, Kaesser UR, Losem CJ. Effects of antihypertensive therapy on hypertensive heart disease. Circulation 1989;80(6 Suppl):IV145.

22. Messerli FH. Left ventricular hypertrophy: Impact of calcium channel blocker therapy. Am J Med 1991;90(5A):27s.

23. Amery A, Birkenhager W, Brixko P, Bulpitt C. Mortality and morbidity results from the European working party on high blood pressure in the elderly trial. Lancet 1985;2:1349.

24. Freis ED. Critique of the clinical importance of diuretic-induced hypokalemia and elevated cholesterol level. Arch Intern Med 1989;149:2640.
25. Heidrich FE, Stergachis A, Gross KM. Diuretic drug use and the risk for hip fracture. Ann Intern Med 1991;115:1.
26. Andersen GS. Atenolol vs bendroflumethiazide in middle aged and elderly hypertensives. Acta Med Scand 1985;218:165.
27. Wikstrand J, Westergren G, Berglund G, et al. Antihypertensive treatment with metoprolol or hydrochlorothiazide in patients age 60–75 years. JAMA 1986;255:1304.
28. Avorn J, Everitt DE, Weiss S. Increased antidepressant use in patients prescribed beta-blockers. JAMA 1986;255:357.
29. Jenkins AC, Knill JR, Dreslinski GR. Captopril in the treatment of elderly hypertensive patients. Arch Intern Med 1985;145:2029.
30. Gibson GR. Enalapril-induced cough. Arch Intern Med 1989;149:2701.
31. The SOLVD Investigators. Effect of enalapril on survival in patients with reduced left ventricular ejection fractions and congestive heart failure. N Engl J Med 1991;325:293.

6

Anticonvulsants

Edward G. Tessier

The incidence of isolated seizure activity and new-onset epilepsy—the chronic condition of recurrent seizure activity—is increased in patients over the age of 60 years (1–3). In the elderly nursing home patient, distinguishing between benign myoclonic jerks (which are associated with central nervous system disorders like dementia and which do not require treatment) and epilepsy is important.

CLASSIFICATION

Accurate classification of seizure type may be helpful in managing seizure activity. Seizures are usually classified as *partial* when they originate in a focal region of the cerebral cortex and *generalized* when they involve both hemispheres of the brain from the onset.

Generalized seizures almost always involve a loss of consciousness; *complex* partial seizures result in altered consciousness whereas *simple* partial seizures do not. The International Classification of Seizure Type is presented in Table 6.1.

CLINICAL PRESENTATION

Partial complex seizure activity may be more prevalent and the clinical presentation is often atypical in older patients (1, 4). Partial complex seizures may be mistaken for confusion, psychosis, or dementia; postictal confusion or paralysis may be prolonged, lasting hours or days, and may be misinterpreted by caregivers as a stroke, delirium, or depression (5).

ETIOLOGY

Determining whether potentially reversible causes are responsible for seizure activity may be helpful for successful treatment. Although up to 70% of older patients have an identifiable cause of seizure activity (3, 6), few etiologies are correctable. Cerebrovascular disease accounts for

Table 6.1.   International League Against Epilepsy—Classification of Epileptic Seizures[a]

I. Partial seizures (focal, local)
  A. Simple partial seizures (consciousness not impaired)
    1. With motor signs
    2. With special sensory symptoms
    3. With autonomic symptoms
    4. With psychological symptoms
  B. Complex partial seizures (with impairment of consciousness)
    1. Simple partial onset followed by impairment of consciousness
    2. With impairment of consciousness at onset
  C. Partial seizures evolving to secondarily generalized seizures
    1. Simple partial seizures (A) evolving to generalized seizures
    2. Complex partial seizures (B) evolving to generalized seizures
    3. Simple partial seizures evolving to complex partial seizures evolving to generalized seizures
II. Generalized seizures (convulsive or nonconvulsive)
  A. Absence
    1. Typical
    2. Atypical
  B. Myoclonic
  C. Clonic
  D. Tonic
  E. Tonic-clonic
  F. Atonic
III. Unclassified seizures

---

[a]Adapted from Proposal for revised clinical and electroencephalographic classification of epileptic seizures: from the commission on classification and terminology of the International League Against Epilepsy. Epilepsia 1981;22:489.

approximately 30% of seizure activity in elder patients; tumors account for about 15%, Alzheimer's disease for approximately 10%, metabolic abnormalities and trauma about 5–7% each, and approximately 30% of seizures are of undetermined etiology (4) (Table 6.2).

TREATMENT

For some patients with new onset seizure activity, correction of the precipitating or etiological factor(s) associated with seizure activity, e.g., elimination of toxins or correction of metabolic abnormalities, is sufficient. Anticonvulsant therapy may be indicated if no correctable metabolic, toxic, or self-limited cause is identified.

Table 6.2. Associations with Seizure Activity

Metabolic	Hypoglycemia	Hypocalcemia
	Hyponatremia	Hypomagnesemia
	Acidosis	Alkalosis
Toxic	Rapid Drug Withdrawal	
	Anticonvulsants	Benzodiazepines
	Alcohol	Barbiturates
	Psychotropics	
	Phenothiazines[a]	Tricyclic Antidepressants
	especially Chlorpromazine	Bupropion
	Promazine	Maprotiline
	Triflupromazine	Amphetamine
	Lithium salts	
	Antimicrobials	
	Penicillins	Enoxacin
	especially Imipenem/cilastatin	Isoniazid
	Chloroquine	Cycloserine
	Ciprofloxacin	Pyramethamine
	Analgesics	
	Meperidine	Propoxyphene
	Fentanyl/sufentanyl	Salicylates
	Mefenamic acid	
	Cardiac Drugs	Verapamil
	Digoxin	Methyldopa
	Lidocaine	Tocainide
	Mexiletine	
	Other	
	Theophylline	Busulphan
	Chlorambucil	Methotrexate
	Radiologic contrast agents	Vaccines
	Illicit drugs	Alcohol
	Rarely	
	Carbamazepine	Phenytoin
Pathologic	Cerebral infarcts	Intracranial bleeds
	Intracranial infections	Head trauma
	Fever	Brain tumor
Psychosocial[b]	Sleep deprivation	Emotional stress
	Strobe lights	

[a]From Cold JA, Wells BG, Froemming JH. Seizure activity associated with antipsychotic therapy. DICP Ann Pharmacother 1990;24:601.
[b]From Chadwick D, Reynolds EH. When do epileptic patients need treatment? Starting and stopping medication. Br Med J 1985;290:1885.

Guidelines

1. *Anticonvulsants should not be used prophylactically in patients who have not previously had a seizure.* The prophylactic use of anticonvulsants in stroke or even in newly diagnosed intracerebral malignancy is not beneficial unless the patient develops actual seizure activity (7). Similarly, prophylactic anticonvulsant use for patients with severe head trauma beyond 7 days does not reduce seizure risk (8).

2. *Drug therapy is most beneficial in patients with recurrent seizures.* Although the utility of initiating anticonvulsants after only one seizure is controversial (9–12), a conservative approach that withholds chronic anticonvulsant use until a clear indication for therapy is present is favored. The literature supporting the utility of drug therapy indicates that therapy should be limited to patients with a seizure focus on EEG, progressive chronic cerebral disorders, or for patients in whom the risk of seizures is particularly great. In patients with recurrent seizures, however, anticonvulsant therapy is usually beneficial (13, 14).

3. *If possible, choose anticonvulsants on the basis of seizure type and drug side-effect profile.* The goal of anticonvulsant drug therapy is to prevent seizures with minimal adverse effects. Simple partial, complex partial, and generalized tonic/clonic seizure types are usually responsive to carbamazepine or phenytoin. Phenytoin should generally be avoided in patients with absence seizures, as it often worsens control of this seizure type. For mixed seizure types, which include absence seizures, valproic acid or divalproex is an appropriate alternative. Carbamazepine and valproic acid have also demonstrated some beneficial effects in patients with manic or bipolar disorders (15–18); thus, for patients with cyclic affective disorders and a seizure history, carbamazepine or valproic acid may do "double duty." Phenobarbital and primidone should be avoided because of their sedating effects.

    There is, however, a growing body of opinion, to which we subscribe, that therapeutic response to anticonvulsants is not predictable, and choice in the elderly should be based on side-effect profile as much as seizure type. All anticonvulsants have significant and hazardous adverse effects, including central nervous system

Contrary to past prescribing practices, multiple-drug regimens are rarely more effective than single-drug therapy and are associated with greatly increased toxicity.

toxicities and bone marrow suppression. Choice of agent must be made, in part, based on individual risk factors for each patient. Common adverse effects are noted in Table 6.3.

4. *Conduct an adequate trial of a single agent before adding a second drug.* An adequate trial of an anticonvulsant involves the use of the agent at doses that produce a therapeutic level for a period of time sufficient to assess efficacy. Treatment failure is often related to use of subtherapeutic doses or to premature discontinuation of the drug. Achieving adequate drug levels with minimal toxicity is more difficult in the elderly, and requires consideration of the pharmacokinetic subtleties of anticonvulsant therapy in the older patient.

5. *Avoid multiple-drug regimens.* Multiple-drug therapy should be limited to patients who fail an adequate trial of two different single agents. Contrary to past prescribing practices, multiple-drug regimens are rarely more effective than single-drug therapy and are associated with greatly increased toxicity.

6. *Be alert to the potential for significant drug interactions.* Carbamazepine, phenytoin, and phenobarbital are potent enzyme inducers and can significantly affect the hepatic clearance of a number of drugs. In a recent listing of the 40 most clinically important drug-drug interactions, anticonvulsants were involved in 25% of the categories listed (19).

Awareness of drug interactions is imperative when discontinuing anticonvulsants as well as adding them to the drug regimen (20, 21). Valproic acid has a lower drug interaction profile and may be useful in long-term care patients with complicated drug regimens. Several clinically important drug interactions are listed in Table 6.3.

7. *Use the lowest dose of anticonvulsants that prevents seizures.* Because of the pharmacokinetic and pharmacodynamic changes in the elderly,

Table 6.3. Commonly Used Anticonvulsants: Implications for Elders

Drug	Seizure Type	Dosage	Drug Interactions[a]	Adverse Effects	Comments
Phenytoin (Dilantin)	Generalized tonic-clonic Simple partial Complex partial (May worsen absence)	200–300 mg/day Occasionally up to 400 mg/day	Major clinical significance Concurrent use may result in *increased* phenytoin levels Chloramphenicol, disulfiram, isoniazid Moderate clinical significance Concurrent use may result in *increased* phenytoin levels Fluconazole, omeprazole, sulfonamides, tricyclic antidepressants, valproic acid (unbound phenytoin levels) Concurrent use may result in *decreased* phenytoin levels Folic acid, rifampin, salicylates, ? valproic acid (total levels), many enteral feedings Use of phenytoin may result in decreased levels/ response to Corticosteroids, cyclosporin, digitoxin,	Dose-related: Nystagmus, ataxia, diplopia, drowsiness, lethargy, encephalopathy, delirium Idiosyncratic: Rash, gingival hyperplasia, osteomalacia, thrombocytopenia, leukopenia, neuropathy, folate deficiency	100 mg Kapseal = 92 mg Suspension = 92 mg tablet form 90% protein bound; increased free levels with hypoalbuminemia, renal failure Nonlinear dose-dependent hepatic clearance; make dosage adjustments slowly, especially at higher levels Consider Ergocalciferol therapy to reduce risk osteomalacia Lab interference: Reduced T4 levels. Time to steady-state: 7–30+ days

| Carbamaze-pine (Tegretol) | Generalized tonic-clonic Simple partial Complex partial | 200 mg b.i.d. to 400 mg q.i.d. | (?) digoxin, doxycycline, estrogens, furosemide, mebendazole, methadone, primidone (increased conversion to phenobarbital), theophylline, tricyclic antidepressants, thyroid, warfarin (after initial increase) Concurrent use may lead to increased risk osteomalacia Acetazolamide Major clinical significance Concurrent use may result in increased carbamazepine levels Erythromycin, isoniazid, propoxyphene Moderate clinical significance Concurrent use may result in increased carbamazepine levels Cimetidine, danazol Concurrent use may result in decreased carbamazepine levels Phenytoin Use of carbamazepine may result in decreased levels/response to | Dose-related: Drowsiness, nausea, vomiting, SIADH, diplopia Idiosyncratic: Rash, neutropenia (common), agranulocytosis (rare), aggravation CHF/HTN | Autometabolism noted within first few weeks of therapy Suspension more rapidly absorbed; may lead to increased peak levels and more CNS toxicity Initiate therapy slowly Time to steady-state: 2–4 days; 14–21 days for completion of autometabolism |

Table 6.3. Commonly Used Anticonvulsants: Implications for Elders *Continued*

Drug	Seizure Type	Dosage	Drug Interactions[a]	Adverse Effects	Comments
			Corticosteroids, estrogens, haloperidol, imipramine, mebendazole, phenytoin, thyroid, warfarin. Concurrent use *may* lead to neurotoxicity: Lithium		
Valproic Acid (Depakene) Divalproex (Depakote)	Absence, generalized tonic—clonic, Complex partial, myoclonic Atonic	250 mg bid (divalproex) to 500 mg qid	Moderate clinical significance Concurrent use may lead to *increased* free valproic acid Salicylates Concurrent use may lead to *increased* levels/ response to Phenobarbital, phenytoin (free levels)	Dose-related: Sedation, thrombocyto- penia, nausea and vomiting (minimized with divalproex), dementia Idiosyncratic: Hepatotoxicity (rare), elevated ammonia	Reduced hepatic clearance in elders Highly albumin bound; protein binding is saturatable Increased free levels in patient with hypoalbuminemia, renal failure Time to steady-state: 3– 5 days
Phenobarbital	Second-line agent for: Generalized tonic-clonic,	60–200 mg/ day	Major clinical significance Concurrent use may lead to decreased levels/ response	Dose-related: Sedation, confusion, nystagmus,	Increased volume of distribution in elders may significantly increase half-life and

Simple partial, Complex partial

Warfarin
Moderate clinical significance
Concurrent use may lead to *increased* phenobarbital levels
Chloramphenicol, MAO inhibitors, primidone, valproic acid
Concurrent use may lead to *decreased* levels/response to
Acetaminophen, β-adrenergic blockers, corticosteroids, disopyramide, doxycycline, estrogen, meperidine (increased nor-meperidine), methadone, neuroleptics, nifedipine, quinidine, theophylline, tricyclic antidepressants, verapamil

paradoxical hyperexcitability, paradoxical insomnia
Idiosyncratic: Rash, osteomalacia, folate deficiency

risk of hangover effect
Consider Ergocalciferol therapy to reduce risk osteomalacia
Time to steady-state: 14–28 days

°Adapted from Hansten P, Horn J. Drug interactions & updates. Vancouver, WA: Applied Therapeutics, Inc., 1990.

lower doses of anticonvulsants may prevent seizures and avoid toxicity without achieving standard "therapeutic" serum levels of the anticonvulsant.

ANTICONVULSANTS

Phenytoin

Of all anticonvulsants, phenytoin is the most problematic to dose. Reviews in extended care facilities indicate significant variation in phenytoin plasma concentrations with levels below 10 (the lower end of the therapeutic range) or above 20 μg/ml (the upper end of the therapeutic range) observed in the *majority* of patients receiving the drug (22, 23). Appreciation of the nature of absorption, distribution, and hepatic clearance is imperative in achieving seizure control without toxicity.

Important issues for the oral absorption of phenytoin include choice of dosage form, timing of dosage, and drug-drug/drug-food interactions. Phenytoin extended-release capsules (Dilantin Kapseals) contain 92 mg of phenytoin acid per 100-mg capsule; the suspension and prompt release forms contain 100 mg of phenytoin acid per 100 mg labeled product. This represents a difference in potency of 24 mg per 300 mg dosage, which may be clinically significant given the nonlinear pharmacokinetic profile of phenytoin. Concurrently administered enteral feedings may result in reduced absorption of phenytoin suspension (24).

Phenytoin is approximately 90–95% plasma protein bound. In patients with hypoalbuminemia, renal failure with uremia, or in patients receiving salicylates or valproic acid, free concentrations of phenytoin can be significantly elevated. Monitoring of unbound phenytoin concentrations may be beneficial in such patients; alternately, maintenance of standard phenytoin levels between 5 and 10 mg/L may, in fact, be therapeutic for patients receiving other highly protein-bound drugs, patients in renal failure, or with low albumin levels (25).

Hepatic clearance of phenytoin follows a nonlinear profile. As doses are increased, clearance decreases and the elimination half-life increases. Thus, significant drug accumulation can continue for weeks after an increase in dosage, and toxicity may be present at "typical" phenytoin doses of 300–400 mg per day (26).

While a number of sophisticated pharmacokinetic formulae or no-mograms can assist in appropriate phenytoin dosing, most clinicians dose the drug empirically. Particular caution, however, should be exercised with increasing dosage for patients who already have levels in the upper part of the therapeutic range. For such patients, small dosage adjustments (e.g., even increases in the total daily dose as little as 30 mg of the extended sodium capsule or 25 mg of suspension) may cause disproportionate increases in serum drug concentrations, mandating careful follow-up over 2–6 weeks.

Adverse effects for phenytoin include gingival hyperplasia (which may affect denture wear in some patients) and osteomalacia (often prevented with supplemental vitamin D therapy). Other adverse effects are listed in Table 6.3.

Carbamazepine

Carbamazepine (Tegretol) is often a preferable choice over phen-ytoin for elder patients. While mild neutropenia is fairly common, serious bone marrow suppression is extremely rare despite the "black box" warning in the package insert. The most common adverse effects include dizziness, blurred vision, and dose-related lethargy and drowsi-ness, all of which can be minimized by making small incremental increases in dosage when initiating or adjusting therapy. The syndrome of inappropriate antidiuretic hormone (ADH) secretion is fairly fre-quently seen and may be dose related.

A suspension form is available; it is absorbed more quickly than the tablet form and may be associated with more central nervous system (CNS) effects secondary to increased peak levels. Carbamazepine induces its own metabolism; autoinduction is generally complete within the first 2 weeks of therapy (27).

Valproic Acid

Valproic acid may also be a good initial therapy for seizures in the older patient. It is available as a syrup or soft gelatin capsule; the divalproex form is available as an enteric-coated tablet. A sprinkle formulation (Depakote Sprinkle) may be mixed with food. Hepatic clearance of valproic acid appears to be decreased in many older patients

(25). Valproic acid is highly protein bound, but at higher levels (i.e., approximately 100 mg/L) protein binding is saturated. This may predispose elder patients (especially those with hypoalbuminemia) to significant toxicity despite typical "therapeutic" plasma levels. Empiric use of lower doses and maintaining levels in the low-normal range may thus be wise with older patients. Adverse effects include nausea and vomiting (significantly reduced with the divalproex form), and dose-related thrombocytopenia. Fatal hepatotoxicity has reportedly occurred only in pediatric patients.

Phenobarbital

While phenobarbital has been utilized as an anticonvulsant for most of this century, it is generally considered a second-line agent because of sedation. The increased volume of distribution of barbiturates may result in excessive daytime somnolence for many elders, even if dosed once daily at bedtime. Phenobarbital is associated with dose-independent behavioral changes and is more likely to affect vitamin D metabolism increasing the risk for osteomalacia (25).

LABORATORY MONITORING

Anticonvulsant levels can help identify probable causes of toxic symptoms or loss of seizure control, or in evaluating the impact of dosage adjustments. In general, however, dosing decisions should not be based on drug levels alone. Some patients require concentrations in excess of the standard laboratory range for adequate seizure control; a reduction of dose to achieve "therapeutic" levels may result in loss of seizure control and is not warranted in such patients unless toxicity is evidenced. Similarly, "subtherapeutic" levels may effectively prevent seizures in older patients with a lower risk of adverse effects than occurs with "therapeutic" levels.

Anticonvulsant levels should be obtained during the postabsorptive ("trough") stage (usually before first morning dose) and should not be drawn until levels have reached predicted steady-state. Levels drawn shortly after the administration of a dose or prior to achieving steady-state can be misleading. Typical times required to reach steady-state for each drug are listed in Table 6.3.

It may be appropriate to order unbound or free levels of phenytoin for patients in whom a clinical reason exists to suspect increased free levels (e.g., hypoalbuminemia, renal failure, concurrent valproic acid therapy) and toxicity, despite "normal" standard phenytoin levels. Free phenytoin levels are more expensive than standard levels, however, take longer to obtain, and are not necessary in most cases.

WITHDRAWAL OF ANTICONVULSANT THERAPY

Clearly, the benefits of anticonvulsant drug therapy for patients must be measured against the possible risks. In addition to the adverse effects noted in Table 6.3. elder epileptic patients receiving anticonvulsant drug therapy are at greater risk for hip and vertebral fractures. The risk is greatest for females over the age of 75 years (28). Possible reasons for the observed increased fracture risk include anticonvulsant-induced osteomalacia and increased risk for falls secondary to drug toxicity.

Seizure-free patients who have been maintained on higher doses of anticonvulsants may benefit from a reduction in dose, and some may be candidates for withdrawal of anticonvulsant therapy entirely. Patients who were prescribed anticonvulsant therapy after a stroke, whether or not a seizure occurred, are especially appropriate candidates for discontinuation (23). Seizures associated with acute stroke are generally self-limiting, not associated with an increased mortality or worse functional outcome, and are relatively infrequent (29), although are more likely to occur after subarachnoid hemorrhage (30). A subset of stroke patients with persistent uncontrolled seizure activity, however, may develop worsening of stroke sequelae (31). While patients with early seizure activity after stroke may be at increased risk for seizure recurrence (32), there are no data to support the efficacy of anticonvulsant treatment in preventing late seizure activity in this population (25). Likewise, patients with seizures related to head trauma may tolerate withdrawal of anticonvulsants without seizure recurrence (33).

Withdrawal of anticonvulsants in patients with complex partial seizures that are secondarily generalized [up to 20% of elder patients with seizure disorders (2)] may be associated with a higher risk of seizure relapse than other types of seizure disorders (33). Withdrawal of anticonvulsants should be considered for most patients, however, who have been seizure free for 2–4 years and have a normal EEG. For patients on multiple drug therapy, slow reduction and elimination of additional drugs should be achieved first. Of note, discontinuation of one anticonvulsant may result in dramatic increases or decreases in the levels of remaining anticonvulsants (21).

Withdrawal of single-drug therapy should be slow and over a period of at least 6–12 weeks (33). When seizures do recur within a few weeks of anticonvulsant withdrawal, the possibility of withdrawal seizures should be seriously considered. Some suggest that withdrawal of anticonvulsants should be conducted even more slowly, over a period of 6 months or longer, to minimize the chance of withdrawal seizures (34).

References

1. Hauser WA, Kurland LT, The epidemiology of epilepsy in Rochester, Minnesota, 1935 through 1967. Epilepsia 1975;16:1.
2. Luhdorf K, Jensen LK, Plesner AM. Epilepsy in the elderly: incidence, social function, and disability. Epilepsia 1986;27:135.
3. Loiseau J, Loiseau P, Duche B et al. A survey of epileptic disorders in southwest France: seizures in elderly patients. Ann Neurol 1990;27:232.
4. Sanders KM, Murray GB. Geriatric epilepsy: a review. J Geriatr Psychiatry Neurol 1991;4:98.
5. Godfrey JBW. Misleading presentation of epilepsy in elderly people. Age Ageing 1989;18:17.
6. Luhdorf K, Jensen LK, Plesner AM, et al. Etiology of seizures in the elderly. Epilepsia 1986;27:458.
7. Cohen N, Strauss G, Lew R et al. Should prophylactic anticonvulsants by administered to patients with newly-diagnosed cerebral metastases? A retrospective analysis. J Clin Oncol 1988;6:1621.
8. Temkin NR, Dikmen SS, Wilensky AJ, et al. A randomized, double-blind study of phenytoin for the prevention of post-traumatic seizures. N Engl J Med 1990;323: 497.
9. Hauser WA. Should people be treated after a first seizure? Arch Neurol 1986;43:1287.
10. Annegers JF, Shirts SB, Hauser WA, Kurland LT. Risk of recurrence after an initial unprovoked seizure. Epilepsia 1986;27:45.
11. Hart RG, Easton JD. Seizure recurrence after a first unprovoked seizure. Arch Neurol 1986;43:1289.
12. Hachinski V. Management of a first seizure. Arch Neurol 1986;43:1290.
13. Chadwick D, Reynolds EH. When do epileptic patients need treatment? Starting and stopping medication. Br Med J 1985;290:1885.
14. Scheuer ML, Pedley TA. The evaluation and treatment of seizures. N Engl J Med 1990;323:1468.

15. McElroy SL, Pope HG. Use of anticonvulsants in psychiatry: recent advances. Clifton, NJ: Oxford Health Care, 1988.
16. Pope HG, McElroy SL, Keck PE, Hudson JI. Valproate in the treatment of acute mania. Arch Gen Psychiatry 1991;48:62.
17. McElroy SL, Keck PE, Pope HG, Hudson JI. Valproate in the treatment of bipolar disorder: literature review and clinical guidelines. J Clin Psychopharmacol 1992;12:42S.
18. Freeman TW, Clothier JL, Pazzaglia P, et al. A double-blind comparison of valproate and lithium in the treatment of acute mania. Am J Psychiatry 1992;149:108.
19. Hansten PD, Horn JR. The top 40 drug interactions. Drug Interactions Newsletter: A Clinical Perspective and Analysis of Current Developments 1991;11:483.
20. Pisani F, Perucca E, DiPerri R. Clinically relevant anti-epileptic drug interactions. J Int Med Res 1990;18:1.
21. Duncan JS, Patsalos PN, Shorvon, SD. Effects of discontinuation of phenytoin, carbamazepine, and valproate on concomitant antiepileptic medication. Epilepsia 1991;32:101.
22. Mooradian AD, Hernandez L, Tamai IC, Marshall C. Variability of serum phenytoin concentrations in nursing home patients. Arch Intern Med 1989;149:890.
23. Oles KS, Gal P, Penry JK, Tapscott WK. Use of antiepileptic drugs in the elderly population. Public Health Rep 1987;102:335.
24. Haley CJ, Nelson J. Phenytoin-enteral feeding interaction. DICP Ann Pharmacother 1989;23:796.
25. Pugh CB, Garnett WR. Current issues in the treatment of epilepsy. Clin Pharm 1991;10:335.
26. Levine M, Orr J, Chang T. Interindividual variation in the extent and rate of phenytoin accumulation. Ther Drug Monit 1987;9:171.
27. Mikati MA, Browne TR, Collins JF, et al. Time course of carbamazepine autoinduction. Neurology 1989;39:592.
28. Annegers JF, Melton LJ, Sun C, Hauser WA. Risk of age-related fractures in patients with unprovoked seizures. Epilepsia 1989;30:348.
29. Kilpatrick CJ, Davis SM, Tress BM, et al. Epileptic seizures in acute stroke. Arch Neurol 1990;47:157.
30. Kotila M, Waltimo O. Epilepsy after stroke. Epilepsia 1992;33:495.
31. Bogousslavsky J, Martin R, Regli F, et al. Persistent worsening of stroke sequelae after delayed seizures. Arch Neurol 1992;49:385.
32. Kilpatrick CJ, Davis SM, Hopper JL, Rossiter SC. Early seizures after acute stroke—risk of late seizures. Arch Neurol 1992;49:509.
33. Callaghan N, Garrett A, Goggin T. Withdrawal of anticonvulsant drugs in patients free of seizures for two years. N Engl J Med 1988;318:942.
34. Wallis WE. Withdrawal of anticonvulsant drugs in seizure-free epileptic patients. Clin Neuropharmacol 1987;10:423.

7

Sedative Hypnotics and Antipsychotics

Edward G. Tessier

Few issues in the long-term care setting are as emotionally controversial as the use of antipsychotics and sedative hypnotics. Indications for use are frequently unclear, and the possibility that they may be prescribed not for the benefit of patients but for the convenience of staff and providers is always a concern.

About 20% of patients in long-term care are given sedative hypnotics (1, 2), and surveys indicate that antipsychotics are used in 20–40% of patients (1–6). In a review of the use of psychotropics in 112 nursing homes, Beardsley et al. noted that 21% of patients receiving psychotropics did not have a documented psychiatric diagnosis or symptoms that would indicate need for psychotropics (1). In a review of Medicaid claims for Illinois nursing home residents, Buck noted that 60% of patients 65 years and older who received antipsychotic agents had a primary diagnosis other than functional or organic mental illness or mental retardation (2). Svarstad and Mount and others found increased tranquilizer use in facilities with lower staffing and resources (3, 4). This chapter will focus on the appropriate role of sedative hypnotics in the treatment of sleep disorders and of antipsychotics in the management of psychosis, agitated dementia, and maladaptive behaviors. A brief discussion of pending Health Care Financing Administration (HCFA) regulation/interpretive guidelines for sedative hypnotic use and recent regulation regarding antipsychotic drug use in long-term care settings is also included.

SEDATIVE HYPNOTICS IN THE MANAGEMENT OF SLEEP DISORDERS

Disturbances in sleep patterns are common in older patients. Increased sleep latency, increased frequency of wakeful periods, increased stage 1 sleep, decreased Rapid Eye Movement (REM) sleep, and a reduction of the deeper stages 3 and 4 sleep are all noted in older individuals (7–10). Such disturbances may lead to sleep deprivation and increased risk of daytime fatigue, impaired cognitive function, irritability, seizures, and hallucinations (7). Interestingly, 70% of caregivers noted that nocturnal wakefulness and/or nocturnal disruptive behavior were factors in the choice to institutionalize their family member (8). The sleep/wake pattern in the long-term care patient varies with his or her baseline level of cognitive function and physical activity. Not surprisingly, nonambulatory demented or bedridden patients appear to spend a greater portion of the 24-hour day asleep and exhibit more daytime sleeping than ambulatory demented patients or nondemented ambulatory and nonambulatory patients (11). The absence of bright daylight in many long-term care settings may also disrupt the circadian wake/sleep cycle (12).

Sleep disorders may be classified as difficulty in initiation and/or maintaining sleep (generally presenting as insomnia), excessive somnolence, and disturbed sleep-wake cycle. Sleep disorders involving the initiation or maintenance of sleep can be further classified as transient or short-term insomnia (lasting a few days to 3 weeks) and long-term or chronic insomnia (lasting longer than 3 weeks) (13). In the long-term care setting, short-term insomnia is often the result of environmental influences, changes in medical condition, or drug effects. Chronic insomnia in long-term care patients is usually caused by depression or depressive symptoms, anxiety, dementia, chronic sedative/hypnotic use, medical illness, or poor sleep/wake habits. Other causes are outlined in Table 7.1.

Disorders of excessive sleepiness or somnolence in older patients are often related to carryover effects of sedative hypnotics or other sedating drugs. Disturbed sleep-wake cycles are observed in many long-term care patients where daytime stimulation may be minimal or where other patients have disruptive nocturnal behaviors.

The primary treatment of sleep disorders should be directed at addressing correctable causes. This often involves treatment of underlying medical or psychiatric conditions, re-evaluating and revising current drug regimens, or altering the environment when possible. Once correctable factors have been identified and addressed, the patient should be encouraged to establish healthy sleep practices. This may include increasing daytime stimulation and activity, participation in a modest exercise program, or, in the long-term care setting, making a room change away from a disruptive peer.

Table 7.1. Disorders of Initiation or Maintenance of Sleep[a]

Causes	Treatment

Sleep apnea
    Apnea 10 seconds or longer
    Results in increased daytime sedation, increased risk mortality
    More common in males than females
	Weight loss, behavior modification to minimize sleeping on back, acetazolamide, nasal continuous positive airway pressure, upper airway surgery, avoidance of sedative hypnotics or alcohol

Restless leg syndrome Strong urge to move legs before falling asleep results in increased sleep latency	? Benzodiazepines, ? opioids, ? L-dopa[b] ? Avoid tricyclic antidepressants?[c]
Nocturnal myoclonus Periodic leg movements resulting in repeated awakenings throughout night	? Benzodiazepines, ? opioids, ? L-dopa
Medical illness Pain syndromes (including arthritis, neuralgias, malignancies, chronic back pain), congestive heart failure with orthopnea, nocturnal leg cramps associated with renal failure, chronic lung disease	Correct or treat underlying abnormality (e.g., analgesia for pain syndromes, diuretics for congestive heart failure)
Psychiatric illness Depression, mania, anxiety, panic disorder, obsessive-compulsive disorder	Treatment directed against underlying psychiatric disorder
Dementia and delirium Alzheimer's disease, sundowning	Attention to good sleep habits; safe environment
Drug use Theophylline, levodopa, lipophilic β-blockers (especially propranolol, pindolol, metoprolol[d]), amphetamines, methylphenidate, thyroid supplements, diuretics administered late in the day, antipsychotics (akathesia)	Avoid/control for offending drugs

Table 7.1. Disorders of Initiation or Maintenance of Sleep^a Continued

Causes	Treatment
Drug withdrawal	
Benzodiazepines, barbiturates, chloral hydrate	Minimize withdrawal effects with slow taper and/or support
Habits	
Caffeine, alcohol, "night owl" syndrome	Control for habit
Behavioral insomnia	
Learned maladaptive behavior associated with sleep or the sleep environment	Behavioral therapy, encourage good sleep habits, alter environment

aAdapted from Prinz PN, Vitiello MV, Raskind MA, Thorpy MJ. Geriatrics: sleep disorders and aging. N Engl J Med 1990;323:520.
bKaplan B, Mason NA. Levodopa in restless legs syndrome. DICP Ann Pharmacother 1992;26:214.
cRoehrs TA, Roth T. Drugs, sleep disorders, and aging. Clin Geriatr Med 1989;5:395.
dRosen RC, Kostis JB, Taska LS, Holzer BC. Beta-blocker effects on objective and subjective measures of sleep in normotensive male subjects. Sleep Res 1986;15:42.

PRINCIPLES OF DRUG TREATMENT OF INSOMNIA IN LONG-TERM CARE PATIENTS

1. *Address correctable causes of sleep disturbance.* This may include adequate treatment of underlying medical conditions (including depression), avoidance of stimulant drugs, and/or alteration of the environment.
2. *Reserve sedative hypnotic agents for patients with disabling symptoms of insomnia where correctable causes cannot be identified.*
3. *When indicated, consider a 1- or 2-night trial of a short-acting benzodiazepine.* Short-term use of triazolam and temazepam is effective in reducing sleep latency and in increasing total sleep time, are short acting, and produce little hangover effect. Oxazepam and lorazepam, while not marketed as sedative hypnotics, are effective alternatives. Agents with long elimination half-lives (e.g., flurazepam, diazepam) are best avoided in the majority of older patients due to excessive somnolence often observed the following day (Table 7.2).
4. *Use low doses.* Age-related pharmacokinetic and pharmacodynamic differences lead to increased intensity and duration of sedative effect

Table 7.2. Sedative Hypnotic Agents Commonly Used with Elders for the Treatment of Disabling or Short-term Insomnia

Drug	Dose	Elimination Half-life[a]	Comments
Triazolam (Halcion)	0.125 mg	1.5–5.0 hours	Increased risk for: rebound insomnia, ? psychiatric disturbances, early AM insomnia, and next day agitation with chronic dosing; no active metabolite
Temazepam (Restoril)	15 mg	8–38 hours	No active metabolite
Estazolam (Prosom)	0.5–1.0 mg	12–18 hours[b]	? Similar risks as triazolam? Undergoes microsomal oxidation[c]
Flurazepam (Dalmane)	15 mg	74–160 hours (includes active metabolite)	Active metabolites; significant hangover effect with many elders
Lorazepam (Ativan)	0.5–1.0 mg	8–25 hours	No active metabolites
Oxazepam (Serax)	10 mg	5–15 hours	No active metabolites
Diphenhydramine (Benadryl)	12.5–50 mg	8 hours	Not as effective as benzodiazepines; anticholinergic effects may be significant (avoid in patients with dementia/ history delirium, benign prostatic hypertrophy)
Chloral hydrate (Noctec)	250–500 mg	4–10 hours	Tolerance with chronic use; not as effective as benzodiazepines; may increase PT when given with warfarin

[a]Adapted, in part, from American Medical Association Drug Evaluations Subscription. Chicago: American Medical Association 1990; Vol 1, Sec 3, Chap 1.
[b]Gustavson LE, Carrigan PJ. The clinical pharmacokinetics of single dose estazolam. Am J Med 1990;88(Suppl 3A):2.
[c]Abramowicz M, Ed. Estazolam—a new benzodiazepine hypnotic. Med Lett Drug Ther 1991;33;91.

of benzodiazepines in older patients. Geriatric doses are approximately half those of younger patients (13, 14).

5. *Recognize the potential adverse effects of benzodiazepine therapy.* All benzodiazepines produce anterograde amnesia. This may contribute to, or be confused with, dementia in many long-term care patients. Some patients may exhibit paradoxical excitation or frank hallucinations. Triazolam in particular may be associated with more frequent psychiatric disturbances than other agents in this class (15, 16); it is unclear whether this is a drug effect or a withdrawal phenomenon with this ultra short-acting agent, but has prompted removal of the drug from some European markets (17). Changes in cognitive function and an increased risk for falls and hip fractures are associated with benzodiazepines, particularly the longer acting agents (18–20).

6. *Avoid chronic benzodiazepine use to minimize tolerance, rebound insomnia, and withdrawal phenomenon.* Chronic use of benzodiazepines is associated with habituation, and loss of efficacy after 2–4 weeks (13). Early morning insomnia and increased daytime anxiety have been associated with chronic administration (e.g., 1–3 weeks) of triazolam (21, 22). In addition, while rebound insomnia can occur after discontinuation of all benzodiazepines, it occurs sooner and is more dramatic with shorter acting agents, and may be more common with older patients (21). Benzodiazepine withdrawal may also present as confusion or disorientation. Discontinuation of long-term benzodiazepine therapy should occur gradually to minimize the risk of withdrawal effects and seizures.

7. *Establish clear guidelines and limits for benzodiazepine use.* The use of "p.r.n." or "p.r.n. for sleep" orders will be interpreted differently by different nursing staff and may lead to either or both excessive and infrequent use at different times during the month. Variable use of a benzodiazepine may result in daytime somnolence, rebound insomnia, withdrawal agitation, or seizures. Instead, establishing clear criteria and limits for use (e.g., give if still awake at 12 midnight; do not give after 2:00 AM; do not give more than three times per week) minimizes problems related to tolerance and variable or excessive use. Frequent use of benzodiazepine sedative hypnotics may soon be interpreted as unnecessary if pending guidelines for the 1992 HCFA regulations are adopted (23). The implications for noncompliance with HCFA regulations are briefly addressed later in this chapter.

8. *Periodically evaluate the need, efficacy, and risks for adverse effects of benzodiazepine therapy.* Often, insomnia is only a short-term response to an admission into the long-term care facility or to a change in environment or social situation. Long-term sedative hypnotic therapy is rarely indicated or in the overall best interest of the patient.

9. *The risks and benefits of nonbenzodiazepine sedative hypnotics generally do not favor their use.* Antihistamine use, specifically diphenhydramine, has the advantage of no habituation and low cost. Unfortunately, its sedative effect declines with regular use, and anticholinergic side effects may produce delirium, changes in cognitive function, and urinary obstruction in the presence of benign prostatic hypertrophy. Chloral hydrate may be a short-term alternative for some patients, but risks for habituation and early development of tolerance limit its long-term utility. Barbiturates should not be used in elder patients because of habituation, significant paradoxical effects, tolerance, hangover effect, and suppression of REM sleep.

10. *When possible, adjust the environment to the patient's clock—not vice versa.* Many patients need a different sleep/wake cycle than the regimented lifestyle of most long-term care facilities. This may be particularly true for demented patients. Small adjustments in the environment (e.g., provision of a supervised area for "night owls" or allowing a patient to "sleep in" undisturbed until noon) may be a dignified and effective alternative to sedative hypnotic therapy.

ANTIPSYCHOTICS: MANAGEMENT OF PSYCHOSIS, AGITATED DEMENTIA, AND MALADAPTIVE BEHAVIORS

Patients with a primary acute and chronic psychosis, psychosis related to dementia and delirium, or otherwise unexplained serious maladaptive behaviors are often residents in long-term care settings. Problem behaviors, including uncooperativeness, aggression, and wandering are noted in approximately one-quarter of long-term care patients, and appear to be most frequent in patients requiring higher levels of care (24, 25). Such behaviors are disruptive and may interfere with the ability of the long-term care staff to provide good care to the agitated patient as well as to other patients. Historically, antipsychotic drugs have been the mainstay of treatment for many maladaptive behaviors in elderly patients residing in long-term care facilities, but reports of abuse of these agents has prompted regulation that is requiring more careful scrutiny of antipsychotic drug use in these settings (26, 27).

Indications for Antipsychotic Use in Long-term Care Patients

DEMENTIA

Dementia is a highly variable, chronically progressive, and multifaceted disorder with behavioral and functional features in addition to cognitive deterioration (28). Drug toxicity, acute delirium, changes in cardiac function, and infections are some of the causes of agitation or psychotic symptoms in demented patients that must be excluded before drug therapy is initiated. Reviews of neuroleptic use in the treatment of

---

Antipsychotics do not improve the intellectual impairment associated with dementia . . . Nonagitated patients will not benefit from antipsychotics, and may be harmed by this relatively toxic group of drugs.

---

dementia suggest that neuroleptics are moderately effective in treating psychotic and agitated behavior in some, but not all, patients (29–33). Improvement is most likely to be noted in patients with severe initial behavior problems, hallucinations, and delusions. Antipsychotics do not improve the intellectual impairment associated with dementia; these agents may, in fact, be associated with deterioration of cognitive function due to excessive sedation. Nonagitated patients will *not* benefit from antipsychotics, and may be harmed by this relatively toxic group of drugs.

DELIRIUM

Delirium is an acute change in cognitive function that usually involves behavioral disturbance and has an organic basis. The abrupt onset and fluctuation of symptoms distinguish delirium from dementia. Delirium may be caused by cardiac, neurological, or infectious diseases, or may be secondary to drug toxicity or metabolic abnormalities (34). Patients with underlying cognitive impairment, over 80 years of age, or recent fractures may be at highest risk for development of delirium (35). A number of drugs, including H_2-blockers, antiparkinsonian drugs, nonsteroidal anti-inflammatory agents, anticonvulsants, corticosteroids, digoxin, β-adrenergic blockers, and benzodiazepines frequently induce behavioral changes in elderly patients (36). Anticholinergics and drugs with strong anticholinergic properties (antidepressants, antihistamines) may be particularly associated with delirium in older patients (37). Even antibiotics, such as ciprofloxacin or trimethoprim-sulfamethoxazole, have caused delirium in patients with organic brain disease (38). Management is based on the identification of organic cause and supportive treatment. Short- term use of antipsychotics may or may not be useful in managing delirium. Haloperidol is generally considered the first drug of choice due to its low anticholinergic profile and minimal sedation; Mellaril (thioridazine) is useful for patients who require greater sedation. Other drugs used by geriatricians and geropsychiatrists are listed in Table 7.3.

Minimizing Adverse Effects with Antipsychotic Therapy

Elders may be at particular risk for development of many adverse effects from antipsychotic drugs including extrapyramidal effects and tardive dyskinesia.

1. **Extrapyramidal Effects:** Extrapyramidal symptoms (EPS) include tremor, festinating gait, drooling, muscle spasms, jitteriness, and repetitive, rhythmic involuntary movements. High-potency agents like haloperidol and trifluoperazine are more frequently implicated. Symptoms may be independent of dose and generally fall into three broad categories: acute dystonic reactions, pseudoparkinsonian reactions, and akathesia.

   Acute dystonic reactions are sudden in onset, occurring 24–48 hours after the initial administration of the agent. Classic features include torticollis, trismus, oculogyric crisis, and opisthotonus. Dystonic reactions can vary in severity and are often quite painful for the patient. Of concern are patients who may have difficulty in communicating their discomfort. Parenteral diphenhydramine is generally the drug of choice, although other anticholinergics or benzodiazepines may also be effective.

   Pseudoparkinsonian reactions may present as a resting tremor, bradykinesia, cogwheel rigidity, or salivary drooling. Pseudoparkin-

Table 7.3. Commonly Used Antipsychotic Agents in Long-term Care[a]

Drug	Initial Geriatric Dose	EPS	Sedation	Anticholinergic	Comment
Haloperidol (Haldol)	0.25–0.5 mg/day up to 20 mg/day	+ + +	+	+	Few cardiovascular effects; injectable and oral liquid forms available
Thioridazine (Mellaril)	10–25 mg/day up to 400 mg/day	+	+ + +	+ + +	Less EPS, but high anticholinergic effects may limit use; oral liquid form available
Loxapine (Loxitane)	5 mg/day up to 100 mg/day	+ +/+ + +	+/+ +	+/+ +	Injectable and oral liquid forms available
Thiothixene (Navane)	1–2 mg/day up to 30 mg/day	+ + +	+	+	Injectable and oral liquid forms available

[a]Adapted, in part, from American Medical Association Drug Evaluations Subscription. Chicago: American Medical Association 1990. Vol 1, Sec 3, Chap 2.

sonism is surprisingly frequent in older patients treated with neuroleptics, especially in patients with modest parkinsonian features
prior to neuroleptic treatment (38). The age-related decline of
dopamine-containing cells in the substantia nigra may explain why
elders appear to be at greater risk for pseudoparkinsonian symptoms
(39) and tardive dyskinesia (40).

Akathesia presents subjectively as a desire to be in constant
motion and objectively as jiggling of the legs, rocking, or pacing. It is
often mistaken for generalized anxiety, agitated depression, or acute
psychosis with an inappropriate increase in the dosage of the
offending drug. Akathesia may be observed in about 20% of patients
receiving antipsychotic drugs (38, 41). Treatment of akathesia
includes a reduction in dose of the antipsychotic and, perhaps, the
addition of propranolol. (It should be noted that propranolol therapy
may increase levels of the antipsychotic over time.) Antiparkinsonian
agents or benzodiazepines may also be tried.

Prophylactic use of anticholinergic agents with antipsychotics
has been discouraged because of the significant risk for adverse
effects (42). Their use is best limited to patients known to have
historically experienced EPS with antipsychotic agents when initiating therapy or to the treatment of clinically significant extrapyramidal
symptoms. Drug-induced parkinsonism may improve over the first
few months of therapy despite ongoing antipsychotic use; as such,
many patients with early parkinsonian symptoms may benefit from
eventual withdrawal of the anticholinergic therapy (43). Adverse
effects of anticholinergic agents are listed in Table 7.4.

2. **Tardive Dyskinesia:** Tardive dyskinesia (TD) is a movement disorder
   induced by chronic antipsychotic and metoclopramide therapy. All
   currently available antipsychotics, with the exception of clozapine, are
   capable of inducing TD. Approximately 80% of male patients and 95%
   of female patients with TD exhibit facial and/or buccal-lingual dyskinesias. Dyskinesias of the body or limbs are noted in about 35% of TD
   patients. Choreoathetoid movements are more commonly seen in elder
   patients with TD (44). The prevalence of TD in patients with a history
   of chronic antipsychotic use 40–50 years of age is about 18%; for
   patients over the age of 60, the rate rises to 38–46% for males and
   42–54% for females (44). Older patients with affective disorders or who
   display early parkinsonian signs may be at increased risk for TD (45).

Table 7.4. Adverse Effects of Anticholinergic Agents Frequently Observed in Older Patients

Autonomic Nervous System Symptoms	Central Nervous System Symptoms
Gastrointestinal	Confusion
Dry mouth, gastroesophageal reflux, reduced stomach emptying time, constipation	Impaired short-term memory
	Visual illusions
	Hallucinations
	Delirium
Other	
Blurred vision, tachycardia, reduced sweating, urinary retention	

In addition, elder patients may be more likely to develop TD after relatively shorter exposures to antipsychotics (44, 46).

Individual patients may show a broad fluctuation in symptoms over time (47). Reducing doses of antipsychotics may increase symptoms while increasing the dose can result in short-term masking of TD symptoms. There is some indication that drug-free periods may actually pose a greater risk for the development of more severe forms of TD (44). Anticholinergic agents, while improving EPS, often worsen TD symptoms. One of the most broadly utilized rating tools for the assessment of TD is the Abnormal Involuntary Movement Scale (AIMS) developed by the National Institute of Mental Health (48). The AIMS rating tool is fairly well suited to routine clinical monitoring in elder patients, although some degree of cooperation is needed (49–51).

There is no consistently effective treatment for TD; consequently, the use of antipsychotics must be avoided unless absolutely necessary and alternative treatment modalities are unsuccessful or inappropriate. Some have even argued that informed consent may be appropriate for the use of antipsychotics (27, 52), although this is, at present, an uncommon practice in many long-term care facilities (53) and may greatly complicate treatment of elderly patients. While symptoms of TD with older patients are less likely to resolve upon discontinuation (54), favorable outcome can occur in any age group and long-term outcomes may be improved with lower dose or discontinuation of neuroleptic therapy (52).

3. **Other Adverse Effects:** Other adverse effects that have been attrib-

uted to antipsychotic therapy include anticholinergic effects, tachycardia and cardiac arrhythmias, increased seizure risk, changes in thermoregulation, neuroleptic malignant syndrome, retinopathy, corneal or lenticular deposits, photosensitivity, weight gain, hepatotoxicity, and agranulocytosis. Sedation and orthostatic hypotension are fairly frequently noted and may place the patient at risk for falls and fractures (19). The relative risks of frequently observed side effects of the more commonly used agents are listed in Table 7.3.

REGULATORY ISSUES IN THE USE OF SEDATIVE HYPNOTIC AND ANTIPSYCHOTIC AGENTS IN Long-term CARE SETTINGS

The Health Care Financing Administration (HCFA) of the Department of Health and Human Services has issued finalized regulations for long-term care facilities participating in Medicare and Medicaid programs as part of the 1987 Omnibus Budget Reconciliation Act (26). These regulations, initially appearing in February of 1989 and effective since October 1, 1990 (55), were revolutionary in attempting to assure "proper use of physical restraints and psychoactive medication." Minor revisions to the original regulations have recently appeared and superceded prior regulations as of April 1, 1992 (26). The regulation specifically mandates that antipsychotic drugs are to be administered only after a comprehensive assessment of the resident and only when necessary to treat a specific condition as diagnosed and documented in the clinical record (26). Gradual dosage reductions and behavioral interventions must be attempted in an effort to discontinue antipsychotic therapy unless clinically contraindicated. In addition, use of a sedative hypnotic agent more frequently than 16 days per month, or use in the absence of ruling out treatable causes of sleep disorder may be interpreted as unnecessary drug use under proposed interpretive guidelines of the current regulation (23). Benzodiazepines and other psychopharmacological agents used for agitation or anxiety may also be strictly regulated under additional proposed guidelines (27). Failure to adhere to these regulations may place the long-term care *facility* at risk for losing Medicare and/or Medicaid funding. An outline of these requirements is provided in Table 7.5.

Table 7.5.   HCFA Requirements[a]/Proposed Requirements[b] for Antipsychotic Use in Long-term Care Facilities[c]

Approved indications[a]
1. Schizophrenia
2. Schizoaffective disorder
3. Delusional disorder
4. Psychotic mood disorders (including mania and depression with psychotic features)
5. Acute psychotic episodes
6. Brief reactive psychosis
7. Schizophreniform disorder
8. Atypical psychosis
9. Tourrette's disorder
10. Huntington's disease
11. Organic mental syndromes (including dementia) with associated psychotic and/or agitated features as defined by:
    (a) Specific behaviors (e.g., biting, kicking, scratching) which are quantitatively (e.g., number of episodes) documented by the facility and which cause the resident to:
    • Present a danger to themselves
    • Present a danger to others (including staff) or
    • Actually interfere with staff's ability to provide care, or
    (b) Continuous crying out, screaming, yelling, or pacing if these specific behaviors cause an impairment in functional capacity and if they are quantitatively (e.g., periods of time) documented by the facility, or
    (c) Psychotic symptoms (hallucinations, paranoia, delusions) not exhibited as specific behaviors in (a) and (b) above if these behaviors cause an impairment in functional capacity
12. Short-term (7 days) symptomatic treatment of hiccups, nausea, vomiting, or pruritus

Unapproved indications[a]
1. Wandering
2. Poor self-care
3. Restlessness
4. Impaired memory
5. Anxiety
6. Depression
7. Insomnia
8. Unsociability
9. Indifference to surroundings
10. Fidgeting
11. Nervousness
12. Uncooperativeness
13. Unspecified agitation

Table 7.5.   HCFA Requirements[a]/Proposed Requirements[b] for Antipsychotic Use in Long-term Care Facilities[c] Continued

14. The use of a p.r.n. antipsychotic drug more than five times in any 7-day period without a review of the resident's condition by a physician

Dosage reductions[a]
An attempt at gradual dosage reduction must be made every 6 months after therapy begins; gradual dose reductions are not necessary if within the last 6 months the resident has had a gradual dose reduction and the dose has been reduced to the lowest possible dose to control symptoms

Screening for abnormal involuntary movements[b]
Use of antipsychotic drugs may be [considered] unnecessary without the performance of an abnormal involuntary movement test upon the initiation of the antipsychotic drug and at least every 6 months thereafter

[a]Special Bulletin: "Revision to the 'Indicators' for Surveyor Assessment of the Performance of Drug Regimen Reviews in Long-term Care Facilities." American Society of Consultant Pharmacists. Arlington, VA; September 1990.
[b]Staff draft—for discussion only. Health Care Financing Administration (HCFA)—Interpretive guidelines for unnecessary drugs. Special Bulletin of the American Society of Consultant Pharmacists. Arlington, VA; November 1991.
[c]NOTE: Does not include proposed rules for annual independent geriatric psychopharmacologic review, informed consent, or use of chemical restraints as outlined in Department of Health and Human Services—Health Care Financing Administration 42CFR Parts 418, 440, 441, 482, 483, 488. Medicare and Medicaid Programs; Omnibus Nursing Home Requirements; Proposed Rules. Federal Register February 5, 1992;57(24):4516.

A 24-month review of antipsychotic drug use in 60 nursing homes revealed that half of patients receiving these agents would be considered ineligible under the HCFA regulations (6). Compliance with these regulations will require the physician to work with the long-term care staff in evaluating and documenting the effectiveness of antipsychotic agents when used for patients with organic mental syndromes. This provides the physician, nursing staff, pharmacist, psychologist, speech therapist, occupational therapist, physical therapist, and activity staff the opportunity to improve patient outcomes cooperatively. Involvement of nursing staff, in particular, is pivotal in evaluating and reducing inappropriate antipsychotic drug use effectively (56–57). A proposed approach to achieve this end is described in Table 7.6.

These regulations will undoubtedly prompt clinicians to seek alternative means to manage agitation and disruptive behaviors in long-term

Table 7.6.   Steps in the Evaluation of Antipsychotic Medication Use in LTC Settings

Action	Responsible Individuals
1. Identify the negative symptom(s) or target (maladaptive) behavior(s) in question (e.g., kicking, screaming, etc.)	MD, RN, psychologist
2. Determine if maladaptive behavior presents a risk for health or safety of resident, other residents, or staff; if behavior interferes with staff's ability to provide care; if behavior/symptom causes patient frightful distress, or impairs patients functional capacity	MD, RN
3. *Determine whether there is a correctable organic basis* for maladaptive behavior (e.g., urinary tract infection, pain, adverse drug effect, etc.); if so, treat appropriately	MD, RN, RPh (for adverse drug reactions)
4. *Determine whether there is a correctable environmental basis* for maladaptive behavior (e.g., is maladaptive behavior a means for the patient to communicate needs or frustrations or gain attention?); if so, adjust environment appropriately	MD, RN, psychologist, speech therapist
5. Determine whether formal psychiatric evaluation is appropriate	MD
6. *If antipsychotic therapy is indicated, begin with low doses and make dosage increases slowly;* antipsychotics are lipid soluble and have long elimination half-lives in older patients; metabolites of chlorpromazine, thioridazine, and loxapine are pharmacologically active and may account for extended activity[a] or toxicity[b]; lower doses are usually effective and are associated with fewer adverse consequences; typical doses in elderly patients are one-third to one-half of those used by younger patients[c]; for patients with maladaptive or combative behavior coexistent with dementia, very low doses are often effective	MD
7. *Establish an ongoing means to document response* to antipsychotic medication; a fairly simple patient-specific checklist of maladaptive behaviors that can be completed on a shift by shift basis will probably suffice; staff compliance with a more complicated data collection system will probably be low; examples of forms adapted for this purpose have been published elsewhere[d,e]	MD, RN, psychologist, RPh

Table 7.6.   Steps in the Evaluation of Antipsychotic Medication Use in LTC Settings *Continued*

Action	Responsible Individuals
8. *Periodically review response* to therapy, attempting slow reductions in dosage to determine lowest effective dose when possible; determine whether environmental manipulations are effective	MD, RN, RPh, psychologist
9. *Evaluate patient for adverse effects,* especially extrapyramidal effects upon initiation of therapy and during the first 2 weeks after dosage increases; screen patients for tardive dyskinesia prior to initiation of antipsychotics and every 3–6 months thereafter; monitor for other adverse effects, including sedation, ocular opacities, anticholinergic and cardiovascular effects	MD, RN, RPh, PT

[a]Cohen BM, Sommer BR. Metabolism of thioridazine in the elderly. J Clin Psychopharmacol 1988;8:336.
[b]Ciccia S, Garattini S. Formation of active metabolites of psychotropic drugs: an updated review of their significance. Clin Pharmacokinet 1990;18:434.
[c]American Medical Association Drug Evaluations Subscription. Chicago: American Medical Association. 1990; Vol 1, Sec 3, Chap 2.
[d]Williams R. Antipsychotic monitoring systems and procedures. Consult Pharm 1990;5:469.
[e]Kalies RF, Muhich M. Effectiveness of a behavior modification medication monitoring system. Consult Pharm 1990;5:531.

care patients. Alternatives may include the use of β-adrenergic blockers, calcium channel-blockers, carbamazepine, lithium, or antidepressant therapy (31). Unfortunately, their use has not been extensively studied in agitated patients with dementia. Nonpharmacological interventions include behavioral management and alterations in the environment; these avenues should be given serious consideration prior to the implementation of pharmacotherapy (58).

References

1. Beardsley RS, Larson DB, Burns BJ, et al. Prescribing of psychotropics in elderly nursing home patients. J Am Geriatr Soc 1989;37:327.
2. Buck JA. Psychotropic drug practice in nursing homes. J Am Geriatr Soc 1988;36:409.
3. Svarstad BL, Mount JK. Nursing home resources and tranquilizer use among the institutionalized elderly. J Am Geriatr Soc 1991;39:869.
4. Nagle B, Pulliam CP. Nursing homes and tranquilizer use among the institutionalized elderly. J Am Geriatr Soc 1992;40:296.

5. Ray WA, Federspiel CF, Schaffner W. A study of antipsychotic drug use in nursing homes: epidemiologic evidence suggesting misuse. Am J Public Health 1980;70:485.

6. Garrard J, Makris L, Dunham T, et al. Evaluation of neuroleptic drug use by nursing home elderly under proposed medicare and medicaid regulations. JAMA 1991;265:463.

7. Haponik EF. Disordered sleep in the elderly. In: Hazzard WR, Andres R, Bierman EL, Blass JP, eds. Principles of geriatric medicine and gerontology, 2nd ed. New York: McGraw-Hill, 1990;1109.

8. Pollak CP, Perlick D. Sleep problems and institutionalization of the elderly. J Geriatr Psychiatry Neurol 1991;4:204.

9. Pressman MR, Fry JM. What is normal sleep in the elderly? Clin Geriatr Med 1988;4:71.

10. Gottlieb GL. Sleep disorders and their management—special considerations in the elderly. Am J Med 1990;88(Suppl 3A):3A-29S.

11. Meguro K, Ueda M, Yamaguchi T, et al. Disturbance in daily sleep/wake patterns in patients with cognitive impairment and decreased daily activity. J Am Geriatr Soc 1990;38:1176.

12. Gillin JC, Byerley WF. The diagnosis and management of insomnia. N Engl J Med 1990;322:239.

13. Gillin JC. The long and short of sleeping pills. N Engl J Med 1991;324:1735.

14. Greenblatt DJ, Harmatz JS, Shapiro L, et al. Sensitivity to triazolam in the elderly. N Engl J Med 1991;324:1691.

15. Oswald I. Triazolam syndrome 10 years on. Lancet 1989;2:451.

16. Bixler EO, Kales A, Manfredi RL et al. Next-day memory impairment with triazolam use. Lancet 1991;337:827.

17. Perry PJ, Smith DA. Triazolam—the never-ending story. DICP Ann Pharmacother 1991;25:1263.

18. Kruse WHH. Problems and pitfalls in the use of benzodiazepines in the elderly. Drug Saf 1990;5:328.

19. Ray WA, Griffin MR, Schaffner W, et al. Psychotropic drug use and the risk of hip fracture. N Engl J Med 1987;316:363.

20. Ray WA, Griffin MR, Downey W. Benzodiazepines of long and short elimination half-life and the risk of hip fracture. JAMA 1989;262:3303.

21. Gillin JC, Spinweber CL, Johnson LC. Rebound insomnia: a critical review. J Clin Psychopharmacol 1989;9:161.

22. Morgan K. Hypnotics in the elderly—what cause for concern? Drugs 1990;40:688.

23. Staff draft—for discussion only. Health Care Financing Administration (HCFA)—Interpretive guidelines for unnecessary drugs. Special Bulletin of the American Society of Consultant Pharmacists. Arlington, VA; November, 1991.

24. Rockwood K, Stolee P, Robertson D. The prevalence of problem behaviour in elderly residents of long-term care institutions. Can J Public Health 1989;80:302.

25. Rovner BW, Steele CD, German P, et al. Psychiatric diagnosis and uncooperative behavior in nursing homes. J Geriatr Psychiatry Neurol 1992;5:102.

26. Department of Health and Human Services—Health Care Financing Administration

42CFR part 431, et al. Medicare and Medicaid; requirements for long-term care facilities and nurse aide training and competency evaluation programs; final rules. Fed Reg 1991;56:48825.

27. Department of Health and Human Services—Health Care Financing Administration 42CFR parts 418, 440, 441, 482, 483, 488. Medicare and Medicaid Programs; Omnibus Nursing Home Requirements; Proposed Rules. Fed Reg 1992;57:4516.

28. Maletta GJ. Treatment considerations in dementing illness. Clin Geriatr Med 1988;4:699.

29. Rosen J, Bohon S, Gershon S. Antipsychotics in the elderly. Acta Psychiatr Scand 1990;83(Suppl 358):170.

30. Phillipson M, Moranville JT, Jeste DV, Harris MJ. Antipsychotics. Clin Geriatr Med 1990;6:411.

31. Wragg RE, Jeste DV. Neuroleptics and alternative treatments—management of behavioral symptoms and psychosis in Alzheimer's disease and related conditions. Psychiatr Clin North Am 1988;11:195.

32. Schneider LS, Pollock VE, Lyness SA. A meta-analysis of controlled trials of neuroleptic treatment in dementia. J Am Geriatr Soc 1990;38:553.

33. Helms PM. Efficacy of antipsychotics in the treatment of the behavioral complications of dementia: a review of the literature. J Am Geriatr Soc 1985;33:206.

34. Beresin EV. Delirium in the elderly. J Geriatr Psychiatry Neurol 1988;1:127.

35. Schor JD, Levkoff SE, Lipsitz LA, et al. Risk factors for delirium in hospitalized elderly. JAMA 1992;267:827.

36. Wood KA, Harris MJ, Morreale A, Rizos AL. Drug-induced psychosis and depression in the elderly. Psychiatr Clin North Am 1988;11:167.

37. Lipowski ZJ. Delirium in the elderly patient. N Engl J Med 1989;320:578.

38. Ganzini L, Heintz R, Hoffman WF, et al. Acute extrapyramidal syndromes in neuroleptic-treated elders: a pilot study. J Geriatr Psychiatry Neurol 1991;4:222.

39. Coffey DJ. Disorders of movement in aging. Semin Neurol 1989;9:46.

40. McDaniel KD, Kazee AM, Eskin TA, Hamill RW. Tardive dyskinesia in Alzheimer's disease: clinical features and neuropathologic correlates. J Geriatr Psychiatry Neurol 1991;4:79.

41. Adler LA, Angrist B, Reiter S, Rotrosen J. Neuroleptic-induced akathisia: a review. Psychopharmacology 1989;97:1.

42. Bohacek N, Bolwig T, Bunney WE, et al. Prophylactic use of anticholinergics in patients on long-term neuroleptic treatment—a consensus statement of the World Health Organization. Br J Psychiatry 1990;156:412.

43. Barnes TRE. Comment on the WHO consensus statement. Br J Psychiatry 1990;156:413.

44. Yassa R, Nair NPV, Iskandar H, Swartz G. Factors in the development of severe forms of tardive dyskinesia. Am J Psychiatry 1990;147:1156.

45. Saltz BL, Ooerner MG, Kane JM, et al. Prospective study of tardive dyskinesia incidence in the elderly. JAMA 1991;266:2404.

46. Yassa R, Nair V, Schwartz G. Early versus late onset psychosis and tardive dyskinesia. Biol Psychiatry 1986;21:1291.

47. Bergen JA, Eyland EA, Campbell JA, et al. The course of tardive dyskinesia in patients on long-term neuroleptics. Br J Psychiatry 1989;154:523.
48. Guy W. Early clinical drug evaluation unit assessment manual for psychopharmacology, Washington, DC: U.S. Department of Health, Education and Welfare,1976;534.
49. Schooler NR. Evaluation of drug-related movement disorders in the aged. Psychopharmacol Bull 1988;24:603.
50. Munetz MR, Benjamin S. Who should perform the AIMS examination? Hosp Community Psychiatry 1990;41:912.
51. Ahrens TN, Sramek JJ, Herrera JM, et al. Pharmacy-based screening program for tardive dyskinesia. DICP Ann Pharmacother 1988;22:205.
52. Casey DE. Tardive dyskinesia. West J Med 1990;153:535.
53. Gurian BS, Baker EH, Jacobson S, et al. Informed consent for neuroleptics with elderly patients in two settings. J Am Geriatr Soc 1990;38:37.
54. Smith JM, Baldessarini RJ. Changes in prevalence, severity and recovery in tardive dyskinesia with age. Arch Gen Psychiatry 1980;37:1368.
55. Department of Health and Human Services—Health Care Financing Administration 42CFR part 405, et al. Medicare and Medicaid; requirements for long-term care facilities; final rule with request for comments. Fed Reg 1989;54.
56. O'Brien J, Doane KW, Risse SC, Bell RA. Reduction of neuroleptic drug use in nursing homes through nursing-oriented pharmacy consultation. Consult Pharm 1991;6:538.
57. Feinberg JL. Non-pharmacologic alternatives to chemical restraints. Consult Pharm 1990;5:370.
58. Jencks SF, Clauser SB. Managing behavior problems in nursing homes. JAMA 1991;265:502.

8

Treatment of Constipation

Edward G. Tessier

Factors predisposing long-term care patients to constipation include reduced or limited mobility, concurrent medication use, and a high propensity for past laxative abuse. Constipation and fecal impaction are frequent problems for a large number of long-term care patients (1). It is not surprising, therefore, that laxative use is widespread in patients who reside in nursing homes (2).

DEFINITION

Constipation can be defined either in terms of frequency of bowel movements or consistency of stool. Patients who have fewer than three bowel movements per week, experience difficulty passing stool due to poor colonic or anorectal tone, or have hard stool consistency can functionally be considered constipated. The perceptions of constipation by the patients, however, are often at odds with those of clinicians—many patients perceive that they are constipated if they do not have a daily bowel movement (3). Such misconceptions have contributed to laxative misuse and widespread overuse among older patients.

PREDISPOSING FACTORS

Age-related physiological changes in colonic and anorectal function vary from person to person, but gastrointestinal transit times are prolonged in most long-term care patients (4). A reduction in the anorectal squeeze pressure (5), and rectal elasticity is observed in older patients, while subjective sensation of rectal volume is generally maintained (6). Impairment in the sensation of rectal vault fullness may be noted, however, in patients with spinal cord lesions or those with cognitive impairments (7), an important consideration for long-term care clinicians.

Problems associated with age-related changes, such as physical inactivity, impairment, medication, decreased intake of high-fiber foods, and perhaps, low fluid intake, play the most significant roles in the etiology of constipation in long-term care patients. Skeletal muscles of the abdominal wall, pelvic floor, and diaphragm assist in normal evacuation; as such, general debility, physical frailty, and inactivity, and neuromuscular disorders including Parkinson's disease or multiple sclerosis contribute to the development of constipation (7). Chronic diseases such as diabetes mellitus, which affects the autonomic function of the bowel, impair bowel function more directly.

Immobility appears to be a particularly important risk factor—bedridden patients are much more likely to develop constipation than ambulatory patients (1). Constipation is also associated with psychiatric disorders such as depression and psychosis, although the association may, in some cases, be a secondary one. Chronic dehydration could lead to constipation because of reduced thirst sensation and impaired renal mechanisms to conserve salt and water (8), diuretic use, and impaired physical or cognitive function that limits free access to fluids. Impaired physical or cognitive function may also contribute to missed cues to defecate, reduce access to regular toileting opportunities, or make it difficult for patients to communicate the need to defecate.

A list of medications whose use can lead to constipation is presented in Table 8.1. Opiates, anticholinergics, chronic abuse of stimulant laxatives, and iron salts, in particular, predispose to constipation.

COMPLICATIONS OF CONSTIPATION

The most important complication of constipation is fecal impaction, which may present in obscure clinical guises. Subtle clues to fecal impaction include a low-grade fever, chest or abdominal pain, leukocytosis, dysuria or anuria, urinary incontinence, or shortness of breath (9). Cognitively impaired patients with impaction may have paradoxical diarrhea or fecal incontinence from continuous seepage of stool, which may predispose bedridden patients to infected decubiti or urinary tract infections (7). Life-threatening complications such as bowel obstruction, perforation, or volvulus may result from unrecognized impaction. Minor complications of chronic constipation include aggravation of hemorrhoids and development of anal fissures related to the passage of hard stools.

Table 8.1.   Drugs Predisposing to Constipation or Fecal Impaction in Long-term Care Patients

Anticholinergics	Narcotic analgesics
Drugs with anticholinergic properties	Diuretics
Antidepressants (especially	Cardiovascular drugs
amitriptyline)	Calcium channel-blockers (especially
Antihistamines	verapamil)
Neuroleptics (especially thioridazine,	α-Adrenergics (e.g., clonidine)
mesoridazine)	Long-term stimulant laxative use
Calcium salts	Bulk laxatives with inadequate fluids
Aluminum salts (including sucralfate)	
Iron salts	

MANAGEMENT

Assessment

While most long-term care facilities document bowel movements each shift, such logs are often inaccurate (4), especially for patients who may self-toilet. In addition, information on stool consistency or difficulty in passing stool is often lacking. Assessment is best made by physical examination, patient report, and direct discussion with nursing and health care staff. Screening for anorectal cancer, by testing for occult blood, and fecal impaction, by digital rectal examination, should always be done.

Identification of Correctable Causes

Drug therapy is the most important correctable contributing cause to constipation in long-term care patients (Table 8.1). Adjusting drug regimens or eliminating incriminating drugs is often a helpful adjunctive measure even if it does not eliminate constipation. Noting other predisposing factors described above may be helpful, as well.

Nondrug Interventions

Establish a "bowel regimen" that includes timed toileting opportunities (especially after meals), and a diet including adequate fluids and fiber. Adding a modest exercise program or increasing physical activity is also helpful.

Drug Therapy

Laxative therapy is reserved for severe or chronic constipation, or for intermittent constipation not responsive to nondrug interventions. Some clinicians routinely use bulk laxatives prophylactically in long-term care, although there are no data to support this practice. Laxatives are classified according to mode of action and include bulk laxatives, emollients, saline, hyperosmotic, and stimulant laxatives. We recommend a stepped approach starting with bulk laxatives.

LAXATIVES

Bulk Laxatives

High-fiber-containing bulk laxatives are not absorbed; they act by osmotically drawing water into the stool to increase stool mass and provide a softer consistency. Additional fluid intake is essential for effectiveness. While bulk laxatives are usually considered safe, they should be used cautiously, if at all, in patients with significant autonomic dysfunction (including stroke or Parkinson's patients), who are predisposed to obstruction or volvulus (10). Some patients complain of

---

While bulk laxatives are usually considered safe, they should be used cautiously, if at all, in patients with significant autonomic dysfunction . . .

---

abdominal bloating or flatulence; high-fiber dietary products such as bran are more likely to cause gas. Bulk laxatives may require up to 3 days to be effective.

Emollients or Stool Softeners

These agents act as surfactants, to increase water content of the stool. Docusate salts generally appear to be safe, but efficacy has been questioned (11). They are often used in hospitalized patients such as those with cardiac disease who should not strain during bowel movement. Like bulk laxatives, docusate may require 72 hours for effect. Docusate may be added to rectal retention enema solutions to assist in the evacuation of

Table 8.2.   Laxative Options for Long-term Care Patients

Class Agent	Dose	Onset of Action	Indication	Cautions
Bulk				
Psyllium (Metamucil, many others)	1 teaspoon qday to TID	24–72 hours	First-line laxative therapy for most patients	Requires additional fluid intake (8–16 oz per dose); avoid if risk for obstruction; cannot be given by NG tube
Unifiber	1–2 tablespoonfuls qday to b.i.d.			Requires additional fluid intake (8–16 oz per dose) Avoid if risk for obstruction; may be given via nasogastric or gastric tube
Bran				May be more likely to cause bloating and gas
Emollient				
Docusate sodium (Colace) Docusate calcium (Surfak) Docusate potassium (Dialose)	100 mg qday up to 240 mg b.i.d. May also be added to rectal enema	24–72 hours	Hard stools Patients with hemorrhoids, fissures Patients who should avoid straining at stool	

Mineral oil	15–45 ml	6–8 hours	Best avoided in long-term care patients	*High risk for aspiration pneumonitis if cognitive or swallowing deficit or if bedridden; may reduce fat soluble vitamin absorption. Avoid dosing with docusate (results in increased mineral oil absorption)
Saline				
Magnesium hydroxide (MOM)	15–60 ml/day	4–6 hours	May be ideal for constipated patients needing antacid	Avoid in patients with renal insufficiency (increased risk hypermagnesemia)
Magnesium citrate	4–10 oz/dose	30–90 minutes		Avoid chronic use
Sodium phosphate/ sodium biphosphate rectal solution (Fleet enema)	4 oz/dose	2–5 minutes	Treatment impaction; management of patients with megacolon	Avoid in renal failure (increased phosphate) and congestive heart failure (increased sodium)

Table 8.2. Laxative Options for Long-term Care Patients *Continued*

Class Agent	Dose	Onset of Action	Indication	Cautions
Hyperosmotic Lactulose (Chronulac)	15–60 ml/day	24–48 hours		Sweet taste; relatively expensive compared to other choices; may cause bloating
Polyethylene glycol and sodium sulfate (GoLytely, Colyte)	1–4 L total given slowly	0.5–8 hours	Prior to radiographic evaluation or to treat impaction	Excessive fluid may be problematic for patients with renal failure or congestive heart failure, or syndrome of inappropriate ADH secretion
Glycerine rectal suppository		15–60 minutes	As part of p.r.n. treatment plan	May cause rectal irritation
Stimulant Bisacodyl (Dulcolax)	5 mg po 10 mg pr	6–12 hours	Patients receiving opiates for terminal pain management	Do not crush oral tablet or dose with antacids, MOM, or milk (will result in upper GI distress); rectal form may cause local irritation
Senna extract (Senokot, others)	Varies	6–12 hours		
Casanthranol (in Peri-Colace, others)	Varies	6–12 hours		

hard stool. The oral liquid form of docusate is particularly unpalatable; use should be limited to administration by nasogastric or gastric tube.

Mineral oil, while effective as a colonic lubricant, poses a particular risk for aspiration pneumonitis in long-term care patients and should not be used in patients who are bedridden, have difficulty swallowing, or have cognitive deficits. Mineral oil should not be used concurrently with docusate to avoid significant systemic absorption of mineral oil. Chronic use of mineral oil may lead to reduced absorption of fat-soluble vitamins.

Saline Laxatives

Magnesium and phosphate salts are generally poorly absorbed and act by increasing osmotic intraluminal pressure, drawing fluid into the colon. Magnesium hydroxide and magnesium citrate are the most commonly used agents in this class; given orally, they act fairly quickly (usually in 30 minutes to 6 hours). Magnesium citrate is probably too irritating for regular use and may result in excessive fluid loss in patients predisposed to dehydration. Magnesium salts may accumulate in patients with renal insufficiency and should, therefore, be avoided.

Sodium phosphate and sodium biphosphate salts are available in a rectal solution form (Fleet Enema) that is often effective in disimpaction. Regular use of enemas may be necessary for managing patients with megacolon (12). They may cause irritation to the rectal mucosa, however, especially in patients with inflamed hemorrhoids. Sodium phosphate/diphosphate enemas contain considerable sodium and phosphate loads and should be used cautiously in patients with congestive heart failure, renal insufficiency, uncontrolled hypertension, or significant edema.

Hyperosmotic Laxatives

Hyperosmotic agents, like saline laxatives, act to draw additional fluid into the colon. Lactulose is the most commonly used agent in this class; it is a nondigestible disaccharide that decreases colonic pH and is used to reduce ammonia levels in patients with hepatic encephalopathy. Its sweet taste is appealing to some patients and unpleasant for others; it is more expensive than alternative laxatives and has demonstrated only modest efficacy in long-term care patients (4).

Glycerine rectal suppositories act osmotically to draw fluid into the rectal vault and also may stimulate the rectal sphincter. They may cause rectal burning, especially in patients with hemorrhoids.

Stimulant Laxatives

Stimulant laxatives increase colonic motility through stimulation of the mesenteric plexuses. Agents in this class include phenolphthalein, aloe, cascara extracts, senna extracts, and bisacodyl. Unfortunately, these agents can cause permanent damage to the mesenteric plexuses when used regularly, which accounts for much of the laxative dependance observed with many older long-term care patients.

Agents in this class should generally be reserved for patients who do not respond to agents listed above. They may be required, however, for patients with autonomic dysfunction and for patients receiving high-dose opiates for terminal pain management. Bisacodyl oral tablets are enteric coated; they should not be crushed or administered with milk of magnesia, antacids, or milk because this may result in significant gastric discomfort.

References

1. Kinnunen O. Study of constipation in a geriatric hospital, day hospital, old people's home and at home. Aging 1991;3:161.
2. Shipp L, Saffles J. An analysis of laxative use in extended care facilities. Contemp Pharm Pract 1979;2:206.
3. Whitehead WE, Drinkwater D, Cheskin LJ, et al. Constipation in the elderly living at home: definition, prevalence, and relationship to lifestyle and health status. J Am Geriatr Soc 1989;37:423.
4. Brocklehurst JC, Kirkland JL, Martin J, Ashford J. Constipation in longstay elderly patients: its treatment and prevention by lactulose, poloxalkol-dihydroxyanthroquinolone and phosphate enemas. Gerontology 1983;29:181.
5. Laurberg S, Swash M. Effects of aging on the anorectal sphincters and their innervation. Dis Colon Rectum 1989;32:737.
6. Altman DF. Changes in gastrointestinal, pancreatic, biliary, and hepatic function with aging. Gastroenterol Clin North Am 1990;19:227.
7. Wrenn K. Fecal impaction. N Engl J Med 1989;321:658.
8. Rolls BJ, Phillips PA. Aging and disturbances of thirst and fluid balance. Nutr Rev 1990;48:137.
9. Gorbien MJ. Constipation in the elderly: the Sepulveda GRECC method no. 34. Geriatr Med Today 1988;7:53.
10. Castle SC. Constipation: endemic in the elderly? Gerontopathophysiology, evaluation and management. Med Clin North Am 1989;73:1497.
11. Castle S, Samuelson M, Cantrell M, Istael D. The efficacy of prophylactic docusate therapy in institutionalized geriatric patients. J Am Geriat Soc 1988;36:586 (Abstract).
12. Wald A. Constipation and fecal incontinence in the elderly. Gastroenterol Clin North Am 1990;19:405.

9

Drug Therapy of Urinary Incontinence

Penny Lamhut

Urinary incontinence in nursing homes has substantial medical, psychological, social, and economic consequences. Incontinence and cognitive impairment are the two main reasons for placement of previously independent elders in long-term care facilities. As many as 50% of all nursing home residents suffer from urinary incontinence (1, 2). Annual health care costs related to urinary incontinence in nursing homes are estimated to be close to $2 billion (3).

TYPES OF INCONTINENCE

There are four basic types of urinary incontinence. Patients in long-term care facilities, however, rarely have a single mechanism underlying their incontinence, which complicates the assessment and treatment of their incontinence. Nevertheless, it is important to understand the mechanisms responsible for their incontinence so that an effective treatment plan can be formulated.

Urge Incontinence

The most common type of urinary incontinence in the elderly is urge incontinence, which is caused by involuntary contractions of the detrusor muscle of the bladder. This often results from defects in the central nervous system (CNS) regulation of the bladder as seen in patients with stroke, Parkinson's disease, and Alzheimer's disease. Hyperexcitability of the sensory pathways of the bladder as a result of infections, fecal impaction, uterine prolapse, benign prostatic hypertrophy, or bladder tumors, and deconditioned voiding reflexes can also lead to detrusor instability and urge incontinence.

Recently, a phenomenon known as detrusor hyperactivity with impaired contractile function has been identified and described (4). This abnormality occurs in a subset of patients with involuntary detrusor contractions. The bladder contracts involuntarily but because of diminished detrusor contractile function, the bladder empties ineffectively. In such cases, a significant amount of residual urine may be present.

Stress Incontinence

Stress incontinence in elderly women develops when anatomic changes affecting the urethrovesical angle cause a weakness of the pelvic floor. Clinically, patients complain of loss of urine with increases in intra-abdominal pressure as occurs with coughing, sneezing, and laughing. A weakness of the internal urethral sphincter can also lead to stress incontinence. The strength of the internal sphincter may be weakened by prostatectomy or as a result of atrophy of the urethra due to postmenopausal estrogen-dependent mucosal changes.

Overflow Incontinence

The two major categories of overflow incontinence are: *(a)* obstruction of urinary outflow and *(b)* atony of the bladder. Obstruction is most frequently caused by benign prostatic hypertrophy, prostatic cancer, and urethral strictures and leads to urinary retention and overflow leakage of urine. An atonic bladder that is unable to empty properly is commonly a result of diabetic autonomic neuropathy. Lower motor neuron disease, alcoholic neuropathy, spinal cord disease, detrusor-sphincteric dyssynergy, and medications may also cause overflow incontinence as a result of bladder atony.

Functional Incontinence

Patients in long-term care facilities often have both physical and cognitive impairments that make it difficult for them to get to the toilet. Incontinence due to the inability or unwillingness to get to the toilet is termed functional incontinence. Elevation of the side rails and use of restraints, for example, renders many patients who would otherwise be able to toilet themselves incontinent. Iatrogenic functional incontinence may also be caused by medications such as diuretics, anticholinergics, psychotropics, narcotics, α-adrenergic blockers and agonists, and β-adrenergic agonists.

EVALUATION

Cure of urinary incontinence in nursing home patients is not possible in most cases. However, improvements can be achieved with appropriate assessment and interventions (5). Urinary incontinence should be evaluated in the majority of patients to maximize benefit from treatment although severely ill or bed-bound patients are unlikely to benefit from evaluation or treatment. Palliative care should be offered to these patients. Their incontinence can best be managed with diapers or, as a last resort, a chronic indwelling catheter.

Evaluation begins with a search for potential underlying conditions that contribute to incontinence. A neurological examination may reveal evidence of a previous stroke or undiagnosed Parkinson's disease. A bimanual pelvic examination should be performed to identify the presence of uterine prolapse, vaginal atrophy, a cystocele or a rectocele. Fecal impaction needs to be ruled out. Evaluation of cognitive function will help identify patients in whom functional incontinence plays an important role. An assessment of the musculoskeletal system and gait will provide invaluable information regarding a patient's ability to get to, and on and off of the toilet.

A urinalysis and urine cultures should be done and postvoid residuals must be measured. An elevated postvoid residual of greater than 100 ml is indicative of overflow incontinence due to obstruction or an atonic bladder. If the urine culture reveals the presence of bacteriuria, a trial of antibiotic treatment for incontinent patients is worthwhile, even if they are

---

. . . postvoid residuals must be measured.

---

asymptomatic. If no improvement is seen following a course of antibiotic treatment, however, further antibiotic therapy will not be helpful.

Routine baseline laboratory studies including electrolytes, creatinine, and glucose are recommended. Urine cytology should also be sent if malignancy is suspected.

Routine formal urodynamic evaluation is expensive, invasive, and frequently not feasible in long-term care patients with multiple disabilities. Multichannel cystometry and uroflowmetry, however, can be useful when the initial evaluation gives uncertain results, when surgery is considered, or when empiric therapy has failed. Despite recent recommendations for more extensive urodynamic evaluations, simple bedside cystometry usually provides sufficient information in debilitated nursing home patients to guide therapy (6).

Bedside cystometry is performed by inserting a single-lumen catheter into the bladder, obtaining a postvoid residual (and urine specimen if not previously collected). Postvoid residuals greater than 100 ml indicate obstruction, bladder atony, or dyssynergy. The bladder is then slowly filled by gravity with sterile water using a 50- to 60-ml catheter tip syringe with the piston removed. The 50-ml mark on the syringe should be held 15-cm above the symphysis pubis. As the bladder is filled, the patient is asked to cough to try to elicit an involuntary detrusor contraction. Record if there is any resistance to filling, the volume at which the first urge to void is perceived, the volume at which the patient feels the absolute need to void, the maximum volume the patient is able to hold, and the volume at which an involuntary detrusor contraction occurs. If the bladder is able to hold greater than 600 ml of fluid without a sense of fullness, diminished bladder sensation is probably present. An involuntary contraction is detected by a 10- to 15-ml rise in the fluid column or by leakage of fluid around the catheter. If no contractions are elicited with the patient in the supine position, after bladder capacity has been reached, various stress maneuvers can be performed to document the presence of stress incontinence. Have the patient stand, if possible, and observe for leakage for 15–30 seconds. If no leakage is observed, ask the patient to cough. Leakage with these maneuvers suggests stress incontinence.

Many functionally or cognitively impaired patients cannot cooperate with all the maneuvers described previously. Nevertheless, bedside cystometry is easily performed and an incomplete evaluation can still provide useful information with regard to the presence of uninhibited detrusor contractions. Bedside cystometry can be done by trained non-physician health care providers and takes about 10–15 minutes to perform.

The clinical evaluation is usually sufficient to establish an initial working diagnosis. The previously recommended evaluation should be tailored to each particular patient. Pre-existing medical conditions, level of functioning, quality of life, and patient and family wishes need to be taken into consideration when deciding on an appropriate therapeutic plan.

TREATMENT

Whenever possible, treatment of urinary incontinence should be based on the underlying pathophysiology and type of incontinence as revealed by the evaluation described previously. In patients residing in long-term care institutions, however, the cause of the incontinence is often multifactorial. Table 9.1 outlines the treatment options for the various types of incontinence.

Table 9.1.   Treatment Options for Urinary Incontinence

Urge incontinence
  Anticholinergic/antispasmodic drugs
    Oxybutynin, 2.5–5.0 mg t.i.d.
    Imipramine, 10–25 mg t.i.d.
  Bladder training
  Surgical removal of obstruction or other irritating pathological lesions
  Estrogens (if atrophic vaginitis or urethritis is present)
  Electrical stimulation
Overflow incontinence
  Surgical removal of obstruction
  Intermittent catheterization
  Indwelling catheterization
  Cholinergic agonists
  α-Adrenergic blockers
Stress incontinence
  Surgery
  Pelvic floor exercises
  α-Adrenergic agonists
  Estrogens
  Biofeedback
  Electrical stimulation
Functional
  Stop drugs with potential adverse effects on continence
  Behavioral therapies
  Incontinence undergarments and pads
  External collection devices
  Environmental manipulations

Table 9.2.   Drugs Used to Treat Urinary Incontinence

Drugs	Dosages	Mechanism of Action	Type of Incontinence
Anticholinergics/ antispasmotics			
Oxybutinin	2.5–5.0 mg t.i.d.	Diminish involuntary detrusor contractions	Urge or mixed (urge and stress) incontinence
Imipramine	10–25 mg t.i.d.		
Propantheline	15–30 mg t.i.d.		
Flavoxate hydrochloride	100–200 mg t.i.d.		
		Increase bladder capacity	
Conjugated estrogens			
Oral	0.625 mg daily	Strengthen periurethral tissues	Stress incontinence
Topical	0.5–1.0 g per application	Decrease inflammation	Urge incontinence with atrophic vaginitis
Cholinergic agents			
Bethanechol chloride	10–30 mg t.i.d.	Stimulate bladder contractions	Overflow incontinence with bladder atony
α-Adrenergic blockers			
Terazosin	1–5 mg daily	Relaxation of urethral sphincter	Overflow incontinence due to BPH
α-Adrenergic agonists			
Imipramine	10–25 mg t.i.d.	Contraction of urethral sphincter	Stress incontinence
Phenylpropanolamine	75 mg b.i.d.		
Pseudophedrine	15–30 mg t.i.d.		

Controlled trials demonstrating significant benefits of pharmacological treatment for urinary incontinence in functionally impaired nursing home patients are lacking (7, 8). Table 9.2 summarizes the drugs available for the treatment of urinary incontinence. Uninhibited detrusor contractions respond to anticholinergic and antispasmotic agents in some patients. Anticholinergic agents block the cholinergic receptors on the detrusor muscle causing an inhibition of bladder contractility, and an increase in bladder capacity and urge threshold. Such agents also cause troublesome and serious side effects associated with their anticholinergic properties that limit their use, including dry mouth, blurred vision, constipation, and confusion. They can also cause urinary retention and, secondarily, urinary tract infections.

Oxybutynin is primarily a muscle relaxant that exerts a direct effect on the smooth muscle of the bladder to prevent involuntary contractions. It also has anticholinergic properties as well and causes the same side effects as other anticholinergic medications. A trial of oxybutynin, 2.5–5.0 mg t.i.d. is reasonable even though there are no studies proving its efficacy in nursing home patients. A postvoid residual should be obtained 2–4 weeks after initiating treatment to identify drug-induced urinary retention.

Imipramine, like oxybutynin, has both antispasmotic and anticholinergic properties. In addition, it exerts an effect on the internal sphincter to increase urethral resistance. Patients with urge incontinence alone or mixed with stress incontinence should be considered for a trial of imipramine in low doses (10–25 mg t.i.d.). It too has substantial side effects, which are discussed elsewhere.

Flavoxate hydrochloride has not been well studied in the elderly and is not recommended for the treatment of urinary incontinence in residents of long-term care facilities. Propantheline has prominent anticholinergic side effects that limit its use in the geriatric population (9). Terodiline, a new drug under investigation possesses both anticholinergic and calcium channel-blocking activity. It has been shown to be effective in suppressing uninhibited detrusor contractions without significant anticholinergic side effects (10). Preliminary studies of other innovative treatments for urge incontinence, such as electrical stimulation, have not been able to demonstrate any beneficial effect in institutionalized patients (11).

Cholinergic agonists and α-adrenergic blockers, such as prazosin, have been used for the treatment of overflow incontinence but their high incidence of side effects and the lack of long-term success argue against their use in this population. Terazosin, a relatively long-acting α-adrenergic blocker that does not cause as much postural hypotension as prazosin, has been used successfully in ambulatory patients for the treatment of urinary retention resulting from benign prostatic hypertrophy. Whether terazosin would be successful in the treatment of overflow incontinence in men residing in long-term care facilities is not known. The lower incidence of adverse side effects suggests that a trial would be reasonable. A therapeutic trial, starting with a dose of 1–2 mg at bedtime, should be continued for several weeks before concluding that it has not been beneficial. It is not known whether chronic therapy is required.

The mainstay of treatment for overflow incontinence is clean intermittent catheterization and toileting regimens. If patients do not tolerate intermittent catheterization and have recurrent urinary tract infections, an indwelling catheter should be reluctantly considered.

Surgery remains the primary treatment of clinically significant stress incontinence. However, because of the other medical problems and functional disabilities of residents in long-term care facilities, surgery is usually not appropriate. In patients with clinically significant atrophic vaginitis, estrogen therapy, either topically or orally, is a reasonable alternative to surgery. Estrogens strengthen periurethral tissues and decrease urethral mucosal irritation. If oral estrogen therapy is given to a woman with a uterus, cyclical progesterone should also be administered. Imipramine is useful in the treatment of stress incontinence especially in cases of mixed stress and urge incontinence. Biofeedback and pelvic floor exercises usually are not feasible treatment options in institutionalized patients with significant cognitive impairment.

In patients with functional incontinence, the underlying physical or psychological disability should be addressed and treated. Analgesics and nonsteroidal anti-inflammatory drugs often provide sufficient pain relief to allow arthritic patients to toilet themselves. Use of diuretics should be critically examined, and other agents substituted when feasible. Caregivers need to provide the patient with access to the toilet or urinal on a regular basis. Restraints should be used only when absolutely necessary for the safety of the patient and staff. Scheduled toileting or inquiry by

Table 9.3. Indications for Chronic Indwelling Catheter

Urinary retention that cannot be surgically corrected and cannot be managed with intermittent catheterization
Skin wounds, pressure sores, or irritations
Comfort of terminally ill or severely debilitated patients

staff every 2 hours may significantly reduce the frequency of incontinence.

Various forms of behavioral therapy have been described in the treatment of all types of urinary incontinence (12–15). Habit training or scheduled toileting consists of taking the patient to the toilet on a regular basis, for example, every 2 hours. With bladder retraining, the interval between trips to the toilet is gradually increased. Prompted voiding regimens incorporates behavioral modification techniques using positive (such as praise or affection) and neutral reinforcements. A great deal of staff time is involved in implementing such behavioral programs. Therefore, this type of treatment should be targeted to those residents most likely to benefit.

The morbidity associated with indwelling catheters does not justify their use unless specific indications exist. Table 9.3 summarizes the major indications for the use of chronic indwelling catheters.

Overall, conventional treatments for urinary incontinence in residents of long-term care facilities are unsatisfactory and new approaches are needed. More critical evaluation of currently available therapies would allow a more rational approach to the treatment of urinary incontinence in long-term care facilities.

References

1. Ouslander JG, Kane RL, Abrass IB. Urinary incontinence in elderly nursing home patients. JAMA 1982;248:1194.
2. Starer P, Liblow LS. Obscuring urinary incontinence: diapering of the elderly. J Am Geriatr Soc 1985;33:842.
3. Hu T. Impact of urinary incontinence on health care costs. J Am Geriatr Soc 1990;38:292.
4. Resnick NM, Yalla SV. Detrusor hyperactivity with impaired contractile function: an unrecognized but common cause of incontinence in elderly patients. JAMA 1987;257:3076.

5. Pannill FC III, Williams TF, Davis R. Evaluation and treatment of urinary incontinence in long term care. J Am Geriatr Soc 1988;36:902.
6. Castleden CM, Duffin HM, Asher MJ. Clinical and urodynamic studies in 100 elderly incontinent patients. Br Med J 1981;282:11.
7. Zorzitto ML, Holliday PJ, Jewitt MAS, Herschorn S, Fernie GR. Oxybutynin chloride for geriatric urinary dysfunction: a double blind placebo-controlled study. Age Ageing 1989;18:195.
8. Ouslander JG, Blaustein J, Connor A, Pitt A. Habit training and oxybutynin for incontinence in nursing home patients: a placebo-controlled trial. J Am Geriatr Soc 1988;36:40.
9. Zorzitto ML, Jewett MAS, Fernie GR, et al. Effectiveness of propantheline bromide in the treatment of geriatric patients with detrusor instability. Neurourol Urodyn 1986;5:133.
10. Tapp A, Fall M, Norgaard J, et al. Terodiline: a dose titrated, multicenter study of the treatment of idiopathic detrusor instability in women. J Urol 1989;142:1027.
11. Lamhut P, Jackson TW, Wall LL. The treatment of urinary incontinence with electrical stimulation in nursing home patients: a pilot study. J Am Geriatr Soc 1991; in press.
12. Hu T, Igou JF, Kaltreider L, et al. A clinical trial of a behavioral therapy to reduce urinary incontinence in nursing homes: outcome and implications. JAMA 1989;261:2656.
13. Hadley EC. Bladder training and related therapies for urinary incontinence in older people. JAMA 1986;256:372.
14. Schnelle JF. Treatment of urinary incontinence in nursing home patients by prompted voiding. J Am Geriatr Soc 1990;38:356.
15. Engel BT, Burgio LD, McCormick KA, et al. Behavioral treatment of incontinence in the long-term care setting. J Am Geriatr Soc 1990;38:361.

10

Cardiovascular Agents

Philip Gaziano

Angina pectoris and congestive heart failure (CHF) are the two major forms of symptomatic heart disease encountered in long-term care. Symptoms of angina in elders do not differ significantly from those encountered in younger patients, although the isolated complaint of dyspnea may occur more frequently as a manifestation of ischemic heart disease, and so-called silent ischemia may be more common in elderly long-term care patients. Response to antianginal therapy is also similar in older and younger patients, although altered pharmacokinetics and pharmacodynamics usually require lower doses or less frequent dosing in the elderly. Choice of therapy is more influenced, however, by comorbid conditions: the presence of chronic lung or hepatic disease may influence the decision to use calcium-blockers rather than β-blockers, or the presence of renal insufficiency may make one reluctant to use angiotensin-converting enzyme (ACE) inhibitors without the opportunity for close monitoring.

CHF, the most common symptomatic cardiovascular syndrome in long-term care, occurs in two clinically distinct forms. Systolic dysfunction, the more common type, is associated with a dilated left ventricle, usually the result of cardiomyopathy or past myocardial infarction (1). It causes the classical signs and symptoms of CHF (2)—an enlarged heart, S3 gallop, edema, and orthopnea. CHF from diastolic dysfunction, on the other hand, is the result of a stiff nondilated left ventricle, often due to left ventricular hypertrophy (LVH), and may not cause typical chronic signs of CHF. Although longstanding hypertension is the major cause of LVH and, hence, the major cause of diastolic dysfunction, angina may cause transient diastolic dysfunction with or without LVH. In addition, LVH may occur in normotensive elderly patients with diffuse atherosclerotic disease, e.g., type II diabetics. Patients with diastolic dysfunction, in contrast to those with CHF from systolic dysfunction, may benefit from therapy that reduces cardiac contractility, blood pressure, or heart rate, such as calcium channel-blockers or even β-blockers.

In contrast to the treatment of symptomatic conditions, treatment of asymptomatic conditions must be approached with great caution in long-term care. Elderly patients have been systematically excluded from most cardiovascular drug trials; as a result, much of the treatment of cardiovascular diseases and symptoms is empirical. Because cardiovascular drugs may have especially serious adverse effects in the elderly, the limited life expectancy of patients in long-term care should be considered when treatment of asymptomatic conditions such as hypertension or prophylactic regimens such as postmyocardial infarction β-blocker therapy that may impair their quality of life are entertained.

Cardiovascular risk factor management in elderly long-term care patients is controversial, because of the uncertain benefits of altering risk factors in the presence of limited life expectancy. There is no doubt, however, that smoking, diabetes, hypertension, and hypercholesterolemia remain major cardiovascular risk factors in the elderly (3), and advanced age itself is an independent risk factor for cerebrovascular disease (4). Of these, only discontinuation of smoking is likely to yield immediate benefit from attention by physicians. Serum cholesterol measurements are of uncertain prognostic value in elderly long-term care patients, and treatment of elevated levels should be conservative, with at least as much concern for quality of life as disease prevention. Treatment of mild-to-moderate asymptomatic hypertension is of doubtful benefit in the very elderly (see Chapter 5), and vigorous control of diabetes can be more harmful than helpful (see Chapter 12).

Electrocardiograms (ECG) are not cost-effective for cardiovascular risk assessment, only rarely identifying occult coronary artery disease, conduction abnormalities, and chamber enlargement. An ECG should be obtained primarily to evaluate cardiac symptoms or as a baseline if cardiac medications are being considered. In most patients the information obtained from echocardiograms, cardiac stress testing, and gaited-blood-pool studies can be obtained with sufficient reliability through bedside clinical observations.

PHARMACOKINETICS AND PHARMACODYNAMICS

The increased total body fat that occurs with aging increases the volume of distribution for the lipophilic β-blockers, such as propranolol, betaxolol, and labetalol, and many of the antiarrhythmics. A longer time or larger than expected loading doses of these medications may be necessary to achieve the desired therapeutic effect, and adverse or therapeutic effects may last longer than expected. On the other hand, decreased total body water reduces the volume of distribution of hydrophilic medications, including cardiac glycosides, the hydrophilic β-blockers such as atenolol, ACE-inhibitors, and calcium channel-blockers, and may lead to overdosing and toxic effects with standard dosing.

Declining renal function is common in elderly patients with heart disease as a result of renovascular disease, and can complicate dosing. Serum creatinine may not accurately reflect renal function as a result of a concomitant decline in muscle mass. The formulas for estimating creatinine clearance in older patients, moreover, assume only a modest decline in muscle mass, and often underestimate renal failure in the severely debilitated or poorly conditioned long-term care patient (5). Medications affected by decreased renal function include digoxin, β-blockers (especially acebutolol, atenolol, and nadolol), many anti-arrhythmics (including tocainide, flecainide, disopyramide, pro-cainamide), and ACE-inhibitors. When adjusting dosing for decreased renal function, longer dose intervals, rather than lower doses, will produce peaks and troughs similar to those of patients with normal renal function.

Dehydration, from a variety of etiologies (6), may cause an exagger-ated response to vasodilation and heart rate reduction, and a dramatic hypotensive response to β-blockers, ACE-inhibitors, calcium channel-blockers, nitrates, antiarrhythmics, narcotics, antihistamines, and phe-nothiazines. Older patients may need fluid replacement that is as vigorous as for younger patients, particularly in the first 24 hours after dehydration (7), although the risk of fluid overload in those with decreased left ventricular (LV) or renal function must be taken into account when estimating fluid maintenance needs.

Pharmacodynamic changes with aging include a blunted bradycardic response to β-blockers and a blunted tachycardic response to β-blockers, which may aggravate or cause postural hypotension. Neurological side effects from cardiovascular drugs such as propranolol may be a reflec-tion of disease- or age-related central nervous system (CNS) changes. Finally, potentially lethal arrhythmias from theophylline and antiarrhythmic agents (e.g., quinidine, procainamide, or digoxin) are also a reflection of age-related and disease-related changes in the way drugs affect the elder's heart. Table 10.1 illustrates the common agents, their indications, and side effects.

CARDIOVASCULAR MEDICATIONS

Digoxin

Digoxin increases the force of atrial and ventricular contraction, and inhibits atrioventricular (A-V) nodal conduction (prolonging its effec-

Table 10.1. Common Cardiovascular Agents[a]

Agent	Angina	Diastolic CHF	Systolic CHF	Side Effects
Digoxin	—	–	0/ +	Nausea, A-V blockade, ventricular ectopia and sudden death
Verapamil	+	+	–	Sinus bradycardia, A-V blockade, hypotension, shock, CHF, constipation
Diltiazem	+	+	–	Sinus bradycardia, A-V blockade, hypotension, shock, CHF, constipation
Nifedipine	+	+	+ /0	Tachycardia, hypotension, peripheral edema
β-blockers	+	+ /0	—	Bronchospasm, A-V blockade, impotence, sinus bradycardia, CHF, depression
Nitrates	+	+	+	Hypotension, rapid tolerance, headache
Diuretics	0	0	+	Hypotension, dehydration, hypokalemia, renal failure
ACE-inhibitors	+	+	+	Hypotension, renal failure, hyperkalemia, cough, + ANA
Morphine	0	+	+	Sedation, hypotension, constipation, respiratory depression

[a]Abbreviations: +, a useful agent; 0, not useful, but not harmful; –, possibly deleterious effects; —, contraindicated.

tive refractory period). When digoxin is used in a patient with near-normal left ventricular function, there is an increase in peripheral vascular resistance that may increase myocardial work and oxygen demand. For this reason, as well as to reduce the risk of lethal ventricular arrhythmias that may lead to an overall increase in mortality, digoxin should never be used unless specifically indicated, and should be discontinued when patients have been taking it chronically without a clear indication, such as atrial fibrillation or end-stage CHF (8).

In the small subset of patients with end-stage CHF that is refractory to afterload reduction alone, digoxin may reduce LV end-diastolic volume, increase cardiac output, and increase renal perfusion. The toxic effects of digoxin, however, make it inappropriate as therapy for chronic compensated CHF if control can be achieved with diuretics and afterload reducers such as ACE-inhibitors, and it should not be used for acute CHF except to control heart rate in rapid atrial fibrillation or flutter.

Digoxin's inhibitory effect on A-V nodal conduction can be helpful in ventricular rate in atrial fibrillation, atrial flutter, or multifocal atrial tachycardia. Heart rate in response to mild exercise is clinically more reliable than serum digoxin levels in assessing efficacy of A-V nodal suppression, and higher than "therapeutic" levels are usually tolerated by patients treated for supraventricular arrhythmias if serum potassium and calcium levels are normal. In general, however, supratherapeutic levels should be avoided in the elderly, because transient changes in renal function or hydration can lead to acute toxicity with little warning. If supraventricular arrhythmias are infrequent or asymptomatic, digoxin is of doubtful benefit and may be harmful.

Digoxin is almost exclusively renally excreted with a half-life of 40 hours in patients with normal renal function, and must be dose-adjusted for renal failure. It should be used with care in patients on calcium channel-blockers (particularly verapamil and diltiazem) or β-blockers, which also slow A-V nodal conduction. Ventricular arrhythmias are an infrequent but serious complication of digoxin's ventricular excitation; the risk of arrhythmias is increased by a low serum potassium or a high calcium, and potassium supplementation should be routinely considered in patients on both digoxin and diuretics.

Calcium Channel-Blockers

VERAPAMIL, (CALAN, ISOPTIN, VERELAN)

Of the calcium channel-blockers, verapamil has the highest selectivity for myocardial calcium channels, while retaining considerable peripheral, predominantly arteriolar activity. Like digoxin, it is useful in the treatment of atrial tachyarrhythmias by slowing atrial and A-V nodal conduction, but unlike digoxin, verapamil also depresses His bundle conduction and depresses rather than enhances ventricular contractility, which may be helpful in the treatment of ventricular arrhythmias. Its direct cardiac suppression reduces myocardial oxygen demand, but may worsen CHF. Verapamil has the longest steady-state half-life which is about 8 hours. It is primarily metabolized in the liver and receives some first pass degradation. It is extensively protein bound and may yield higher serum levels in malnourished patients.

DILTIAZEM (CARDIZEM)

Because it has less affinity for myocardial receptors and higher affinity for peripheral vascular smooth muscle, diltiazem is a little less likely to cause A-V nodal blockade or CHF, but also less likely to be as useful for atrial tachyarrhythmias and ventricular arrhythmias. It undergoes hepatic metabolism, is extensively protein bound, and has a slightly shorter half-life of 5–6 hours.

NIFEDIPINE (PROCARDIA, ADALAT)

With a low affinity for myocardial calcium channels and a strong affinity for peripheral vascular smooth muscle, nifedipine is useful in the treatment of hypertension and angina, as are the others. The relative lack of significant cardiac suppression makes it potentially useful as an afterload reducer in the treatment of acute systolic CHF, but makes it unhelpful in atrial or ventricular arrhythmias. Reflex tachycardia occurs in response to rapid pressure lowering, but less often with sustained-release preparations.

Peripheral edema, which is not usually seen with other calcium channel-blockers, may occur with nifedipine, although less so with sustained-release preparations. A harmless byproduct of the "XL" sustained-release preparation is a "ghost pill," which is excreted in the stool. Nifedipine has the shortest half-life of the calcium channel-blockers, about 3 hours, which does not increase with age, and, like the others, it is extensively protein bound and liver metabolized. Like verapamil, there is significant first pass metabolism by the liver; as a result, sublingual or buccal absorption may produce a quicker onset of action than the 20-minute onset after oral administration, although pharmacologists disagree on this issue. GI absorption is slowed by food.

ADVERSE EFFECTS

In general, calcium channel-blockers are among the safest cardiovascular agents in the elderly population (9, 10). Side effects are caused by calcium channel blockade of gastrointestinal (GI) or genitourinary (GU) smooth muscle and CNS tissue: anorexia, nausea, vomiting, diarrhea, constipation, urinary retention, dizziness, insomnia, somnolence, depression, and headache. Hypotension may occur, especially in the presence of volume or calcium depletion. Verapamil and diltiazem, and, to a lesser degree, nifedipine, can cause heart block or CHF, particularly when used with β-blockers, digoxin, benzodiazepines, tricyclics, other anticholinergic medications, or in the presence of an already impaired myocardium or conduction system potassium depletion, or hypercalcemia. All calcium channel-blockers are available in sustained-release preparations, although the longer half-life medications, such as regular verapamil, may have pharmacokinetics similar to sustained-release preparations in older patients. Tables 10.2 and 10.3 describe the

Table 10.2. Dosing of Selected Calcium Channel-Blockers and Digoxin

Agent	$T_{1/2}$ (hr)	Dosing Range	Comments
Verapamil	8[a]	80–240 mg b.i.d.-t.i.d.	Non-SR preps may be used b.i.d. or qday in the elderly
Diltiazem	6[a]	30–120 mg t.i.d.-q.i.d.	SR dosing is usually b.i.d. or qday in the elderly
Nifedipine	4	10–40 mg t.i.d.-q.i.d.	XL preparations are used qday in the elderly
Digoxin	40[a]	0.1–0.25 mg daily	Must be carefully adjusted for renal function

[a]Increased with age.

Table 10.3. β-Blocker Dosing

Agent	$T_{1/2}$ (hr)	Dosing for Angina[a]
Metoprolol (Lopressor)	3.5	25–50 mg q.i.d./t.i.d.
Labetalol (Normodyne)	4	25–50 mg q.i.d./t.i.d.
Pindolol (Visken)	6	5–10 mg t.i.d./b.i.d.
Atenolol (Tenormin)	7	25–100 mg b.i.d.
Nadolol (Corgard)	16	20–100 mg daily

[a]All β-blockers may be administered qday or b.i.d. for hypertension.

activities of the various calcium channel-blockers compared with each other and to digoxin and β-blockers.

β-Blockers

By reducing oxygen demand and cardiac output, β-blockers are useful in the management of angina and hypertension, and for postmyocardial infarction (MI) care of patients who do not have systolic CHF. β-Blockers are also useful in treating essential tremor, withdrawal syndromes, hyperthyroidism, and to a lesser extent anxiety symptoms.

β-Blockers vary with respect to their half-lives, volumes of distribution, and tissue distributions (which affect their side-effect profiles), drug delivery systems, and cardioselectivity. Figure 10.1 shows their relative water lipid solubilities; the more lipophilic ones cross the blood-brain barrier easily and cause slightly more CNS side effects.

The clinical usefulness of the degree to which a β-blocker can selectively block the cardiac β_1-receptors preferentially over the pulmonary β_2-receptors is controversial: In higher doses, even the cardioselective medications may cause β_2-receptor blockade and bronchospasm. Hence, all β-blockers should be avoided in patients with severe lung disease or bronchospasm.

Unstable angina and MI tend to occur more frequently in the early morning hours just before or at the time of awakening. A long-acting β-blocker, such as atenolol, may be given before bedtime to provide protection in the preawakening hours. Table 10.3 gives common dosing for angina; dosing intervals for hypertension should be longer, rarely more than b.i.d., even for drugs with a short half-life.

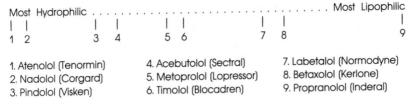

Figure 10.1. Lipophilic and hydrophilic properties of β-blockers.

Nitrates

Nitrates reduce cardiac preload through venodilation, and, to a lesser extent, reduce afterload as a result of arteriolar dilation in higher doses. When given sublingually, the onset of action is within 2 minutes and the duration of action is about 30 minutes, compared with 30 minutes and 3 hours, respectively, for a standard oral dose of isosorbide dinitrate. They are predominantly metabolized in the liver, with a small amount of renal excretion.

Tolerance to nitrates develops very quickly, and hence nitrates are more effective as short-term p.r.n. medications. If used as daily therapy for more than 2 or 3 days, there should be a daily drug-free "washout" time of 10 hours. If the most symptomatic period is at night, for example, topical nitrates may be applied before supper and removed after breakfast.

The major side effect of nitrates is hypotension, although headaches are common. It must also be noted that high venous pressures are needed to overcome dominant right-sided heart failure (rare), and nitrates or other venodilators may severely reduce cardiac output in such patients. The simple maneuver of asking a symptomatic patient to lie flat, which will make a left heart failure temporarily worse but will have little effect on or may even improve right heart failure, can assist in determining whether nitrates may be helpful.

ACE-inhibitors

In patients with chronic CHF, blocking the conversion of angiotensin I to the potent arteriolar vasoconstrictor angiotensin II with an ACE-inhibitor prolongs survival and may dramatically improve symptoms. This effect is seen to a lesser extent with pressure lowering from nitrates (11, 12). In the presence of renovascular disease, particularly but not exclusively with renal artery stenosis, the loss of angiotensin II can cause rapidly progressive renal failure. Since an individual patient's need for angiotensin-mediated renal blood flow regulation cannot be reliably predicted, serum creatinine should be checked before and shortly after starting an ACE-inhibitor, and when dehydration is suspected or likely. Potassium may also rise as a result of the loss of aldosterone effect, and potassium supplements and potassium-sparing agents should be stopped when starting an ACE-inhibitor (1). In diabetic patients, ACE-inhibitors decrease protein excretion, and may thus delay the progression of diabetic renal disease.

Adverse effects include occasional dizziness, headache, and fatigue. Captopril has caused neutropenia, agranulocytosis, and aplastic anemia, mostly in conjunction with high doses and concomitant renal failure or connective tissue diseases. GI and GU side effects are less frequent than with calcium channel-blockers. Because they may cause a rash, fever, positive antinuclear antibody titers, arthritis, and eosinophilia, ACE-inhibitors should not be used in patients with collagen vascular and autoimmune diseases. The annoying cough that may be caused with ACE-inhibitors is believed to be inflammatory in nature; it is not serious, but usually requires discontinuation of medication.

Antiplatelet and Anticoagulant Agents

Warfarin is the most reliable drug for long-term anticoagulation. An active thrombotic process, however, should be treated initially with heparin, which may be given subcutaneously two or three times daily for the first 1 or 2 days, because of an initial prothrombogenic effect of warfarin in some patients. The administration of heparin and warfarin should overlap for 4–5 days. In the elderly, warfarin should be started at a low maintenance dose, without a loading dose.

Warfarin has many important drug interactions. It should not be used with aspirin or other nonsteroidal anti-inflammatory drugs (NSAIDs) that greatly increase the risk of serious or fatal bleeding. It may directly interact with certain antibiotics, and antibiotics such as the third-generation cephalosporins may, in turn, decrease the colonic bacterial production of vitamin K, indirectly predisposing patients to antibiotic-related bleeding. Interactions among the anticonvulsants and warfarin are complex and potentially dangerous: Phenytoin and tegretol increase the metabolism of warfarin, thereby decreasing its anticoagulant effect; warfarin, on the other hand, decreases phenytoin metabolism and increases the amount of free anticonvulsant. When it is necessary to use warfarin and anticonvulsants together, therefore, careful monitoring of anticonvulsant levels and the prothrombin time is essential.

Low-level warfarin anticoagulation provides most of the benefits of aggressive therapy with substantially lower risk. One should aim for a prothrombin time (PT) of only 1.25–1.5 times control (usually 12 seconds) giving PT levels of 15–18 seconds. In some elderly high-risk patients, even levels of 13.4–14.0 seconds (with a control PT of 12) provide adequate therapeutic effect; the PT should never exceed 18 seconds.

Antiplatelet agents are not as effective as anticoagulants at preventing thrombosis, but have fewer side effects and complications. Aspirin is the cheapest and most effective: its effect on platelets is permanent and clinically evident for 8–10 days, or until most of the platelets, which have a 12-day life span, are replaced. The proper dose of aspirin is controversial. Although many clinicians prefer up to two aspirin twice daily, there is no evidence that more than one aspirin per day is required. Even a low-dose "baby" aspirin increases the risk of upper GI bleeding and peptic ulcer disease, but less so than higher doses.

The lack of significant side effects, the ease of administration, and the rapidity (minutes) with which it works make aspirin a consideration for initial treatment of any potential thrombotic process, even before the diagnosis is certain. It may be helpful as prophylaxis in stable angina to reduce the risk of progression to unstable angina and MI, and may reduce thrombotic complications of cerebral and peripheral vascular disease (still a controversial issue after decades of study, however). It may even reduce the risk of colon cancer, although the mechanism is not well understood. NSAIDs have short-term antiplatelet activity and may be used in patients with aspirin intolerance, but must be used in full anti-inflammatory doses (e.g., 1200–1800 mg of ibuprofen daily); thus, they cause greater gastric and renal toxicity than low-dose aspirin.

Ticlopidine is a new potent antiplatelet agent and intermediate strength vasodilator. It has been tested in the elderly, and has significantly fewer GI side effects than aspirin. Although expensive, it may be used for patients who do not respond to or tolerate aspirin (4). It can cause abdominal cramps, diarrhea, and rashes; neutropenia occurs early in therapy and resolves when the drug is discontinued. Dipyridamole (Persantine) is not useful as an antiplatelet agent, despite continued widespread use.

Antiarrhythmic Drugs

β-Blockers and calcium channel-blockers reduce mortality up to 5 years following acute MI, and some of their therapeutic effect is a reduction of sudden death from ventricular arrhythmias (13). Their utility for antiarrhythmic therapy in patients without a recent infarction or unstable coronary artery disease, however, has not been proved. Because these agents should not be used in patients with poor LV function, it was hoped that other antiarrhythmics might provide similar benefit.

. . . antiarrhythmics such as tocainide, flecainide, procainamide, and quinidine have increased rather than decreased mortality in post-MI patients with poor LV function . . .

Unfortunately, antiarrhythmics such as tocainide, flecainide, procainamide, and quinidine have increased rather than decreased mortality in post-MI patients with poor LV function and in those with asymptomatic nonsustained ventricular ectopy (14). They should be used *only* for symptomatic arrhythmias, and only then with the understanding that symptom amelioration is being gained at the risk of serious adverse effects and, possibly, increased mortality. The role for antiarrhythmic therapy, including digoxin, in long-term care patients is very limited, indeed.

References

1. Leibofvitch ER. Congestive heart failure: A current overview. Geriatrics 1991;46:43.
2. Parmley W. Pathophysiology and current therapy of congestive heart failure. J Am Coll Cardiol 1989;13:771.

3. Miller M, Gottlieb S. Preventive maintenance of the aging heart. Geriatrics 1991; 46:22.
4. Adams H, Gordon L. Epidemiology of and stroke-preventive strategies for atherothromboembolic brain infarction in the elderly. Clin Geriatr Med 1991;7:401.
5. Goldberg TH, Finklestein MS. Difficulties in estimating glomerular filtration rate in the elderly. Arch Intern Med 1987;147:1430.
6. Silver AJ. Aging and risks for dehydration. Cleve Clin J Med 1990;57:341.
7. Hoffman N. Dehydration in the elderly: insidious and manageable. Geriatrics 1991;46:35.
8. Packer M. Symposium on therapeutic challenges in the management of congestive heart failure (Parts 1 and 2). J Am Coll Cardiol 1988;12:262, 546.
9. Viddt D, Borazonian R. Calcium channel blockers in geriatric hypertension. Geriatrics 1991;46:28.
10. Ben-Ishay D, Leibel B, Stressman J. Calcium channel blockers in management of hypertension in the elderly. Am J Med 1986;81(Suppl 6A):30.
11. Katz A. Changing strategies in management of heart failure. J Am Coll Cardiol 1989;13:513.
12. Consensus Trial Study group. Effects of enalapril on mortality in severe congestive heart failure. N Engl J Med 1987;316:1429.
13. The Multicenter Diltiazem Postinfarction Trial Research Group. The effect of diltiazem on mortality and reinfarction after reinfarction. N Engl J Med 1988;319:385.
14. Podrid PJ, Levine PA, Klein MP. Effects of age on antiarrhythmic drug efficacy and toxicity. Am J Cardiol 1989;63:735.

11

Pain Management

Philip Gaziano

Perhaps the most subjective of all complaints presented to a physician is pain—the discomfort may represent emotional distress, anxiety, fatigue, loss, loneliness, or the response to a number of noxious sensory stimuli including the stimulation of classic pain nerve fibers. In all of these circumstances, however, the patient's description of pain must be taken seriously as a request for the physician's help.

The clinician's first task, to identify the cause of the discomfort, is made difficult by our limited vocabulary for describing these sensations. The patient may have little insight into the true cause of his or her discomfort, and the caregiver may be hindered by differences in the cultural significance of pain, language barriers, and neurological disabilities such as aphasias. Use of a pain scale such as Katz's ADL index or Lawton's IADL scale (1) may be helpful in assessing and following the patient's pain. A simple 1–10 scale (using a smiling face at one end and a pained face at the other may bypass language barriers) may be preferable to complex ones that may confuse pain with other somatic complaints.

Pain thresholds vary among individuals and circumstances. Some patients complain very little despite what we believe to be great discomfort, and others complain of pain at seemingly minor discomforts. More difficult to understand is variation in complaints in the same individual at different times. We all tolerate pain better when we expect it and are prepared for it, as in the acceptance of muscle discomfort when exercising. But tolerating pain takes energy: Fatigue, illness, anxiety, and other stresses may increase pain because they tax the energy needed to tolerate it. Hence, a change in the pattern of expressed discomfort may represent either a change in an organic cause of pain or a change in the ability to cope with it.

Reducing discomfort, either by reducing or eliminating the cause of pain or by providing ways to cope with it better, has a significant impact on the quality of life. Just as mood can affect pain perception, pain affects mood to the point of causing depression or other psychiatric and nonpsychiatric illnesses. Lessening pain will free psychic resources to be more active and to engage in more enjoyable activities, and the resulting increased mobility may improve the management of other chronic illnesses.

MULTIPLE-DRUG REGIMENS AND THE HAZARDS OF P.R.N. DOSING

The anticipation of pain increases discomfort, by increasing circulating catecholamines that stimulate pain receptors. In addition, forcing patients to delay pain relief by asking for pain medication on a p.r.n. schedule permits the intensity of pain to increase to the point that attempts to regain pain control require increased medication. Requiring patients to request pain medication every 3–4 hours can also create conflicts and mistrust among patients and staff.

Continuous dosing of opiates or nonsteroidal anti-inflammatory drugs (NSAIDs) for expected or chronic pain is always preferable and will provide better pain control at reduced total medication requirements. Omitting scheduled doses if the patient does not need medication or if excessive sedation is noted is more rational than p.r.n. dosing.

Adding another pain medication or nondrug therapy that works by a different mechanism may reduce the total dose of individual drugs. For example, combining an NSAID, heat, massage, and an opiate agonist (or, in chronic pain, adding a low-dose tricyclic; or, in a patient with a

---

. . . forcing patients to delay pain relief by asking for pain medication on a p.r.n. schedule permits the intensity of pain to increase to the point that attempts to regain pain control require increased medication.

---

peripheral neuropathy, adding a low-dose anticonvulsant) can reduce the dose requirements and, hence, the side effects of the individual drugs.

Inflammation that results from tissue trauma may benefit from individual attention for pain control. Hence, use of low-dose (not p.r.n.) NSAIDs with regular heat and massage for 7–10 days, and p.r.n. opiates, particularly at bedtime to ensure sleep for the first few days of discomfort, may provide better pain control, preserve activity, and reduce the total amount of narcotics used.

TREATMENT OF PAIN

Nondrug Therapies

Ice, heat, splinting, bracing, casting, physical therapy, topical anesthetics, and local injections of anesthetics or steroids should be employed whenever possible (2). Ice is of use primarily in injuries of the extremities, within 48 hours of the injury; heat is useful in axial, predominantly back and neck, injuries. There is as much individual variation in the response to local therapy as in the response to pharmacological intervention, so patients' perceptions of the relief afforded should be trusted. Mechanical devices that limit mobility of a painful area may prevent further tissue damage and pain (3).

Telling a patient what to expect, even if it means admitting that their pain may not be completely eliminated, will reduce unrealistic expectations and relieve their anxiety that a serious underlying cause is being missed, or that the staff is neglecting them. Older patients may benefit from counseling and behavioral therapies to modify their response to pain (4), and the use of physical and occupational therapy can reduce the need for medications while reassuring them that function is not lost.

Acetaminophen

Acetaminophen acts peripherally to reduce pain receptor sensitivity, and acts through a direct action on the hypothalamic temperature-regulating centers to provide antipyresis. It has little or no anti-inflammatory activity and fewer adverse effects than NSAIDs. It is rapidly absorbed orally or rectally, takes effect in about 10 minutes, and provides pain relief for approximately 4 hours. Hepatic elimination is not affected by age, but it is slower in patients with liver disease.

Acetaminophen is the safest analgesic for mild, short-duration pain. Only those patients with severe or progressive liver damage, those taking hepatotoxic drugs, such as high doses of zidovudine (AZT), or patients with rare acetaminophen allergies need avoid it. The major disadvantages to its use is its lack of anti-inflammatory activity, which makes it less useful in chronic or immune-mediated pain (5) management, such as in rheumatological diseases, cancer, degenerative diseases, infectious diseases, or trauma. In osteoarthritis, which has a secondary but weak inflammatory component, acetaminophen may be as effective as ibuprofen (6). There is some evidence that slightly higher doses, e.g., 1 g every 4 hours (Extra-strength Tylenol), provide more pain relief than the usual 650-mg dosage.

Acetaminophen-induced hepatic necrosis is dose-dependent and can occur with either a single toxic dose of more than 7.5 g (>30 regular or 20 Extra-strength Tylenol tablets) or chronic doses of 1 g or more over a relatively short period. Irreversible hepatic failure and death rarely occur with an acute dose of ≤ 15 g (45 regular acetaminophen tablets), although toxic doses may be lower in patients with pre-existing liver disease, volume depletion, malnutrition, or concomitant hepatotoxic therapies. Acetylcysteine (Mucomyst) should be promptly administered when intentional or accidental overdosing occurs. Other adverse effects, seen primarily with chronic use, are infrequent, i.e., analgesic nephropathy, discussed later, and hemolytic anemia, which is seen primarily in patients with rheumatological diseases.

Nonsteroidal Anti-inflammatory Agents

Patients over 65 years old (12% of the population) consume 40% of NSAIDs sold (7). Similar to acetaminophen, NSAIDs are centrally acting antipyretics and locally acting analgesics that reduce the sensitivity of pain receptors. But, unlike acetaminophen, they are also potent anti-inflammatory agents that inhibit cyclo-oxygenase, which is needed to convert arachidonic acid into prostaglandins. Prostaglandins, among other actions, stimulate pain receptors, increase vascular permeability, and protect the gastric lining from acid and digestive enzymes (8). Because inflammation plays a major role in most pain syndromes, NSAIDs should be considered as the next treatment option after acetaminophen and local measures. The pain-inducing role of inflammation may be underestimated by clinicians—swelling and redness in a rheumatic or gouty joint is easy to see, but less apparent is the substantial inflammation that may accompany cancer, trauma, infarction, and degenerative diseases and infection.

The major adverse effect of NSAIDs is gastric irritation from loss of the protection of prostaglandins that are normally produced by the gastric lining. The occurrence of gastric irritation is similar among the NSAIDs, although some clinicians believe that the nonacetylated salicylates such as salasate produce less GI toxicity. Overall, incidence of gastric toxicity is low, but increased in the elderly, who are also at risk for fatal silent upper GI hemorrhage (9).

Gastric irritation can be treated or prevented in many patients with concomitant use of misoprostol (Cytotec), a synthetic analog of the protective prostaglandin E_1, or an H_2-antagonist. Fewer than 10% of patients require preventive therapy, although it is prudent in those with a history of gastritis or ulcer disease, or in those who develop symptoms while on therapy.

Analgesic nephropathy, a serious toxicity that occurs fairly commonly with chronic NSAID use, may also rarely occur with acetaminophen or corticosteroids. It is encountered primarily in patients with the types of chronic diseases that are prevalent in elderly long-term care residents—pre-existing renal disease, extensive vascular disease, volume depletion (often from concomitant diuretic use), cirrhosis, CHF, and increasing age, all of which reduce renal blood flow. It is, to some extent, dose related and is reversible. CNS adverse effects include cognitive impairment, psychosis, and aseptic meningitis; they are dose dependent and are also reversible. Aseptic meningitis is seen predominantly in patients with connective tissue diseases, primarily systemic lupus erythematosus (10). True aspirin allergies are rare.

Aspirin is, by far, the least expensive NSAID, followed by generic ibuprofen; proprietary NSAIDs are 3–50 times more expensive. There is no evidence that, in equivalent doses, newer NSAIDs are better at relieving pain or at stopping inflammation than aspirin (9, 11), but some differences are worth noting. The antiplatelet activity of aspirin is irreversible and lasts for the life of the platelet, about 10 days. Thus, aspirin must be avoided in patients taking warfarin or in those who are at risk for bleeding complications. Platelet inhibition produced by other NSAIDs is quantitatively less and briefer in duration.

Nonaspirin NSAIDs have a longer therapeutic effect than aspirin. Most can be routinely dosed t.i.d., and many clinicians begin with b.i.d. dosing in the elderly. Doses required to provide similar 24-hour pain relief with b.i.d.-dosed aspirin or acetaminophen, on the other hand, would produce toxic effects. Naproxen and sulindac (Clinoril) have long half-lives (15–16 hours); a trial of once-daily dosing is reasonable. Dosing shorter half-life NSAIDs b.i.d. such as ibuprofen may also provide 24-hour relief and should be tried; a higher dose of NSAIDs with a longer dosing interval may even be safer than lower doses with shorter dosing intervals. Piroxicam (Feldene), which has a half-life of 2–3 days, should be dosed qday or even every other day.

Nonacetylated salicylates, such as choline magnesium trisalicylate (Trilisate), diflunisal (Dolobid), magnesium salicylate (Magan and others), and salsalate (Disalcid, Salflex) may have less gastric toxicity but they probably also have less anti-inflammatory activity. Because their cyclo-oxygenase activity is somewhat reduced, they can be thought of as intermediate—between acetaminophen and the other NSAIDs, although closer to the NSAIDs. Sulindac (Clinoril) may be less nephrotoxic, and indomethacin may be more nephrotoxic than other NSAIDs.

When changing from one NSAID to another, because of ineffectiveness or adverse reactions, it is usually appropriate to choose one from a different biochemical class of drugs. When using NSAIDs chronically (including aspirin), it is prudent to check hemoglobin, renal function, and stool guaiacs every 3 months. Table 11.1 gives a comparison of common NSAIDs.

Opiate Agonists

Opiates are indicated when acetaminophen or NSAIDs alone are ineffective or cannot be used, such as in the presence of significant liver or kidney disease. Major adverse effects are respiratory depression, constipation, urinary retention, alterations in mental status, and physical dependence or abuse. Most patients tolerate many times the usual analgesic dose without respiratory depression, although they may exhibit changes in the respiratory pattern, such as Cheyne-Stokes respirations—a stable, although abnormal pattern. All of the adverse effects of the opiates are reversible over time, and can be reversed acutely with opiate antagonists such as naloxone (Narcan).

Table 11.1. NSAIDs and Acetaminophen

NSAID Class[a]	Agent (Formulations)	$T_{1/2}$ hours	Average Dose	Analgesic Dose Range
1.	Acetaminophen (325, 500, and 650 mg)	2	650 mg q4h	500–1000 mg q4h
	Aspirin (75, 325, 500, and 650 mg)	1	650 mg q4h	325–1000 mg q4h
2.	Salsalate (Disalcid; 500 and 750 mg)	2	500 mg q6h	500–750 mg q6h
3.	Flurbiprofen (Ansaid; 50 and 100 mg)	6	100 mg q8h	50–100 mg q8h
	Ibuprofen (Motrin; 200, 400, 600, and 800 mg)	2	400 mg q6h	200–800 mg q6–8h
	Naproxen (Naprosyn; 250, 375, and 500 mg)	12	250 mg q8h	250–500 mg q8–12h
4.	Indomethacin (Indocin; 25, 50, and 75 mg)	5	50 mg q8h	25–75 mg q8h
	Sulindac (Clinoril; 150 and 200 mg)	8	150 mg q12h	150–200 mg q12h
	Tolmentin (Tolectin; 200, 400, and 600 mg)	2	400 mg q6h	200–600 mg q6h
5.	Meclofenomate (Meclomen; 50, and 100 mg)	3	50 mg q6h	50–100 mg q6h
6.	Phenylbutazone (Butazolidin; 100 mg)	2	100 mg q6h	100 mg q6–8h
7.	Piroxicam (Feldene; 10 and 20 mg)	48	20 mg q24h	20–40 mg qday
8.	Nabumetone (Relafen; 500 and 750 mg)		1 g q24h	1–2 g q24h

[a]NSAID classes: 1. acetylated salicylates; 2. nonacetylated salicylates; 3. proprionic acids; 4. indole acetic acids; 5. fenamic acids; 6. pyrazoles; 7. oxicams; 8. naphthylacetic acid.

Patients receiving other CNS depressants, such as barbiturates, benzodiazepines, or alcohol; and those with brain stem damage from stroke, encephalopathy, or trauma, or with loss of CO_2 respiratory drive from longstanding COPD, however, may develop significant respiratory depression on even standard doses of opiate agonists. Mental status changes vary widely among individuals, but are less with morphine, which, along with its lower cost and varied routes of administration, makes it the opiate of choice. True dependence is rarely a problem in the long-term care setting, because access to drug can be controlled.

The variety of routes of administration of the opiate agonists facilitate their use in the chronic care setting. Morphine, for example, can be given by the IM, SC, IV, PO, SL, or rectal routes (12), and the combination of parenteral and liquid preparations allows fine-dose adjustments. MS contin provides 12-hour activity with a single PO dose, and comes in many strengths, obviating the need for a continuous drip even in severe cancer pain. A new potentially useful agent not yet well studied in the elderly, is the fentanyl patch (13). Table 11.2 gives a comparison of common opiates, with each column listing approximate equivalent dosing among the different agents, taking morphine as the standard.

Other Agents

Anticonvulsants, such as carbamazepine (Tegretol) and phenytoin (Dilantin), low-dose tricyclic antidepressants (used in one-third to one-half typical doses), and muscle relaxants, such as short-acting benzodiazepines are effective adjuncts in pain control. Anticonvulsants may alleviate peripheral neuropathy pain by affecting pain transmission in the spinal cord (14). Low-dose tricyclics (but not fluoxetine) also seem to reduce spinal cord pain transmission, may reduce the perception of pain, and may reduce the worsening of pain from sleep deprivation (14, 15).

General Guidelines for Pain Management in the Elderly

1. Provide *reassurance* and *realistic expectations*, even if it means admitting that some pain will not be relieved.
2. Use ice, heat, splints, physical and occupational therapy, and

Table 11.2.   Opiate Agonists

Agents (Preparations)	Ratio of Parenteral to PO Strength	Equivalent PO Dosing For		
		Mild Pain	Moderate Pain	Severe Pain
Morphine:[a] (Tabs: 10, 15, and 30 mg) (Rectal suppositories: 5, 10, 20, and 30 mg) [Oral solution: 2, 4, and 20 mg/ml]	4:1	5 mg q4h	10–20 mg q4h	30–40 mg q4h
Morphine SR (MS Contin): (Tabs: 15, 30, 60, 100, and 200 mg)		15 mg q12h	30–60 mg q12h	90–120 mg q12h
Codeine:[a] (Tabs: 15 and 30 mg, or w/ 300–325 mg Tylenol; 7.5, 15, 30, and 60 mg) [Sol: 15 mg/5 ml or 12 mg + 120 mg Tylenol/5 ml]	2:1	15–30 mg q4h	45–60 mg q4h	
Fentanyl (Duragesic); (Topical Patch: 25, 50, 75, and 100 µg/h)			25–50 µg q3day	75–100 µg q3day
Hydromorphone (Dilaudid):[a] (Sol: 1 mg + 100 mg guaifenesin/5 ml) (PO Tabs: 1, 2, 3, and 4 mg) (Rectal Sup: 3 mg)	5:1	1 mg q6h	2–14 mg q6h	6–8 mg q6h
Methadone:[a] (Tabs: 5, 10, and 40 mg) (Sol: 5 and 10 mg/5 ml)	2:1		5–10 mg q6h	15–20 mg q6h
Oxycodone: (Tabs: 5 mg, Sol: 5 mg/5 ml) (Percocet): (5 mg w/325 mg Tylenol) (Percodan): (5 mg w/325 mg aspirin)		5mg q4h	10–15 mg q4h	

[a]Parenteral available

nondrug therapies, when possible, to reduce the need for systemic medication.

3. *Counseling* and behavior modification are useful in the elderly.
4. Acetaminophen is the first p.r.n. choice for short-duration pain not accompanied by inflammation.
5. *NSAIDs* are the first choice for chronic and inflammatory pain syndromes, including those from infection, cancer, infarction, trauma, allergies, and autoimmune or rheumatological disease.
6. Use NSAIDs cautiously in patients with a history of peptic disease or GI bleeding, and consider *gastric protection* with omeprazole, misoprostol, or H_2-blockers.
7. Use NSAIDs and Tylenol with caution in those patients with *suspected low renal perfusion,* such as those with severe systemic vascular disease, low volume states, CHF, ascites, and proteinuria.
8. Check hemoglobin, renal function, and stool guaiacs every 3 months for patients taking NSAIDs chronically.
9. Use *regular, not p.r.n.,* dosing for persistent pain, even if only for a few days.
10. For chronic pain, first try *low-dose NSAIDs* at b.i.d. dosing.
11. Consider increasing the NSAID dose before reducing the dosing interval.
12. Consider *low-dose tricyclic antidepressants* for chronic pain syndromes, especially when accompanied by insomnia, depression, or for fibromyalgia.
13. *Low-dose anticonvulsants* may be useful in pain associated with peripheral neuropathy and spinal cord injuries.
14. Short-acting benzodiazepines are useful for muscle spasm and for related sleep disturbances.
15. *Combining drugs:* NSAIDs, opiates, and tricyclic antidepressants, which act at different sites, reduce adverse effects when used in combination at lower doses.
16. Opiate agonists are under-dosed and underused, but use them cautiously in patients with COPD or CNS disease.
17. Consider using MS Contin or a fentanyl patch in patients with chronic severe pain.

References

1. Pace W. Geriatric assessment in the office setting. Geriatrics 1989;44:29.
2. Ferrer-Brechner T. Anesthetic techniques for the management of cancer pain. Cancer 1989;63:2343.
3. Ferell B. Pain management in the elderly. Geriatr Care Rehabil 1989;3:1.
4. Kwentus J, Harkins S, Lignon N, et al. Current concepts of geriatric pain and its treatment. Geriatrics 1985;4:48.
5. Forman W, Straton M. Current approaches to chronic pain in older patients. Geriatrics 1991;46:47.
6. Bradley J, Brandt K, Katz B, et al. Comparison of an antiinflammatory dose of ibuprofen, an analgesic dose of ibuprofen, and acetaminophen in the treatment of patients with osteoarthritis of the knee. N Engl J Med 1991;325:87.
7. Mazanec D. Conservative treatment of rheumatic disorders in the elderly. Geriatrics 1991;46:41.
8. Hochberg M. NSAIDs: Mechanisms and pathways of action. Hosp Pract 1989;3:185.
9. Griffin M, Ray W, Schaeffer W. Non-steroidal antiinflammatory drug use and death from peptic ulcer in elderly persons. Ann Intern Med 1988;109:359.
10. Hoppmann R, Peden J, Ober S. Central nervous system side effects of nonsteroidal anti-inflammatory drugs. Arch Intern Med 1991;151:1309.
11. Schlegel S, Paulus H. Non-steroidal and analgesic therapy in the elderly. J Clin Rheum Dis 1986;12:245.
12. Pitorak E, Kraus J. Pain control with sublingual morphine. Am J Hospice Palliative Care 1987;3/4:39.
13. Enck R. Transdermal narcotics for pain control. Am J Hospice Palliative Care 1990;7/8:15.
14. Sundaresan N, DiGiacinto G, Hughes J. Neurosurgery in the treatment of cancer pain. Cancer 1989;63:2365.
15. Goldenberg D. Diagnostic and therapeutic challenges of fibromyalgia. Hosp Pract 1989;9:39.

12

Treatment of Type II Diabetes Mellitus

Philip Gaziano

Glucose intolerance increases with age, although it is not clear how much aging itself contributes to the increasing prevalence. Body composition changes (increased fat) and reduced exercise undoubtedly play some role in the development of glucose intolerance in the elderly. The prevalence of diabetes mellitus increases nearly 9-fold from about 2% in persons aged 20–44 years to about 18% in persons 65–74 years old; the prevalence of glucose intolerance is much greater, reaching nearly 41% in persons over the age of 65 years (1).

The criteria for diagnosis of diabetes in older persons have been subject to controversy because the glucose intolerance that develops with aging results in fasting and postprandial glucose concentrations that are higher in the presumably nondiabetic elderly than in younger persons. In general, a fasting blood sugar level above 140 mg/dl or a postprandial sugar above 200 mg/dl is strong evidence for the diagnosis of diabetes in the elderly. Intermediate glucose levels of 120–140 mg/dl fasting, and 140–200 mg/dl postprandial should be viewed suspiciously and repeated. If "disease labeling" is an important issue, a glucose tolerance test may be appropriate for persons with intermediate results; there is no justification, however, for routine glucose tolerance testing for the elderly. Many commonly used drugs affect glucose tolerance (Table 12.1).

Type I diabetes, an autoimmune disease in persons with a genetic predisposition, is rare in the elderly; type II (noninsulin-dependent or adult-onset diabetes) diabetes comprises >90% of elderly diabetics (2–5). A small number of type II diabetics have low insulin production as a result of partial pancreatic destruction from chronic pancreatitis or other causes, but, for most elderly diabetics, insulin resistance is the basis for their hyperglycemia. Type II diabetics produce high basal insulin concentrations, but are less sensitive to the effects of insulin, due both to a reduction in the number of insulin receptors on fat, liver, and muscle cells, as well as reduced insulin activity at these sites. In time,

Table 12.1.   Drugs That Affect Glucose Tolerance*a*

Drugs that can cause hyperglycemia
  Corticosteroids
  Diuretics (thiazides, furosemide, chlorthalidone)
  Estrogens
  Nicotinic acid
  Phenytoin
  Phenothiazines
  Lithium
  Sympathomimetics (albuterol)

Drugs that can cause hypoglycemia
  Alcohol
  β-Blockers
  Coumadin (warfarin)
  MAO inhibitors
  Sulfonamides
  Cimetidine
  Anabolic steroids

*a*From Goldberg et al. Diabetes mellitus in the elderly. In: Hazara WR, Andres R, Bierman EL, Blass JP (eds). Principles of geriatric medicine and gerontology. New York: McGraw-Hill, 1990:739.

insulin receptors on the pancreatic cells are also affected, and islet cells lose some of their ability to produce a postprandial bolus of insulin.

Obesity increases insulin resistance in type II diabetics and nondiabetics; whereas weight loss and exercise reduce insulin resistance, they do not completely reverse it (6). Blood glucose control in type II diabetics is worsened by stress, corticosteroids (endogenous or therapeutic), and immune mediators such as tissue necrosis factor (TNF). Unlike type I diabetics, however, whose metabolic status may rapidly deteriorate despite careful medical management, type II diabetics rarely develop ketoacidosis or hyperosmolar state after recognition and treatment of their disease (7).

THERAPY

Diet

Weight reduction and maintenance of a normal weight is the cornerstone of management of diabetes. Diabetics should eat a balanced diet, one that provides a reliable, constant caloric intake at scheduled times. Special "diabetic" diets are rarely needed in the elderly diabetic. Total caloric intake is more important than the type of diet, and reducing total caloric intake improves glycemic control. Concentrated or large amounts of simple sugars, however, should still be avoided. Dietary intake by confused or ill elderly patients is erratic, and medication adjustment and nasogastric or intravenous fluids and nutrition may be required to prevent hypoglycemia. Exercise, often difficult to achieve for patients in long-term care, may be beneficial, even if limited in intensity, scope, and duration (8).

Sulfonylurea Antihyperglycemics

Sulfonylurea antihyperglycemics improve the sensitivity of insulin receptors to insulin, permitting smaller amounts of insulin to have greater biological activity (9, 10). Type II diabetics should be treated with an oral sulfonylurea if diet, exercise, and weight loss alone do not reduce fasting blood glucose levels below 180–200 mg/dl. Control can be achieved with oral therapy for most elderly type II diabetics, but insulin may be required in about one-third. Reasons for failure to achieve blood sugar control with oral agents include: obesity and inactivity; inadequate doses; use of older, less effective agents; and the occurrence of a short-term stressor, such as a respiratory infection. In addition, drugs such as diuretics, corticosteroids, and β-blockers may worsen blood sugar control or antagonize the therapeutic effects of oral agents.

Oral agents may be grouped into the newer, short-acting drugs, including glyburide and glipizide (Table 12.3), and the older, longer-acting agents, including chlorpropamide, tolazamide, and tolbutamide, which should no longer be used for initial therapy.

Sulfonylureas are primarily metabolized by the liver and excreted in the urine; thus, the duration of their hypoglycemic effect may be prolonged by hepatic or renal failure. Drug interactions with nonsteroidal anti-inflammatory drugs (NSAIDs), warfarin, or β-blockers may enhance their hypoglycemic effects. Their only frequent adverse effect is hypoglycemia, which may be difficult to recognize in the elderly because of their blunted catecholamine response. The older, long-acting oral agents may have a prolonged and dangerous hypoglycemic effect, lasting days.

Table 12.2.   Insulin Action (Hours) After Subcutaneous Administration

Type of Insulin	Onset	Peak	Duration
Short-acting			
Insulin (regular)	½	3	6
Prompt insulin zinc (Semilente)	1	5	12
Intermediate-acting			
Insulin zinc (Lente)	2	10	20
Isophane insulin (NPH)	2	10	20

As with insulin, dosing of oral agents must be individualized according to blood sugar control. Initial doses should be low, however, because some elderly patients are very sensitive to the hypoglycemic effect of sulfonylureas. The usual starting regimen for glipizide (Glucotrol) or glyburide (Diabeta, Micronase) is 2.5 mg daily with breakfast with weekly increases to a dose of 10 mg or until fasting blood sugars are below 200 mg/dl. If fasting sugars are still unacceptably elevated, an afternoon dose should be added, until a total daily dose of 20–30 mg for glyburide or 30–40 mg of glipizide is reached.

It is prudent to attempt to achieve control slowly, over a period of several months in elderly type II diabetics—hypoglycemia from aggressive treatment is far more hazardous than brief periods of hyperglycemia (11,12). A goal of fasting blood sugars between 100 and 150 mg/dl is preferable to tighter control below 100 mg/dl, and fasting blood sugars of 200 mg/dl may be safer for elderly patients whose activity and dietary intake fluctuate widely. The lack of convincing evidence that tight

. . . in elderly Type II diabetics—hypoglycemia from aggressive treatment is far more hazardous than brief periods of hyperglycemia.

glucose control reduces the vascular or neurological complications in the elderly type II diabetic further argues for conservative, rather than aggressive treatment of hyperglycemia.

Table 12.3. Oral Antihyperglycemics

Agent	Half-life	Duration of Effect	Starting Dose	Maximum Daily dose
Glyburide (DiaBeta, Micronase)	2 hr	16–24 hr	2.5 mg daily	30 mg/day (10 mg t.i.d.)
Glipizide (Glucotrol)	4 hr	12–18 hr	2.5 mg daily	40 mg/day (20 mg b.i.d.)

Insulin in Type II Diabetics

While still controversial, adding insulin to maximal oral therapy in type II diabetics, rather than substituting insulin for sulfonylureas if control is not satisfactory, has potential advantages (9, 10, 13). The concomitant use of sulfonylurea agents may allow reduced insulin dosing and, if the reasons for poor control are obesity or a concurrent stress, withdrawal of insulin after weight loss or treatment of stresses is facilitated.

Adding insulin to oral agents should be considered if fasting blood sugar levels remain above 150 mg/dl, or if 11:00 AM (just before lunch) or 4:00 PM (just before dinner) blood sugar levels are above 250 mg/dl. A 7:00 AM subcutaneous 5-unit dose of human intermediate acting (Humulin NPH or lente) insulin may be initiated, and slowly increased until either the 4:00 PM or fasting sugar level is below 150 mg/dl. If the 4:00 PM blood sugar level is less than 150 mg/dl, but the 11:00 AM sugar levels remain high, 5 units of regular (short-acting) human insulin may be added to the 7:00 AM NPH/lente; it may be necessary to reduce the 7:00 AM NPH/lente insulin dose if addition of regular insulin causes the 4:00 PM glucose level to fall below 120 mg/dl. Afternoon, "split dose" insulin should be avoided if possible to minimize the risk of nocturnal hypoglycemia. Table 12.2 gives a comparison of the most commonly used human insulins.

Withdrawal of Insulin

Elderly patients assumed to be insulin dependent may have been started on insulin during a period of physiological stress, or may not have had an adequate trial of full doses of the newer oral agents. Because of the weight loss that occurs with advanced age, some diabetics who were started on insulin when they could not be controlled with oral therapy may no longer require insulin in their later years.

Type II diabetics treated with doses of up to 40 units of insulin may respond to oral agents alone, especially if the new regimen is combined with weight loss and moderate exercise (8). Patients receiving less than 20 units of insulin can discontinue insulin without tapering, and begin taking a daily dose of 5 mg of glyburide or glipizide. Patients receiving 20–40 units of insulin daily should have stepwise reduction of their insulin while adding 5 mg of glipizide or glyburide and adjusting the dose of oral agent. During stress or infection, insulin may be temporarily required, but the oral agent should usually be continued to facilitate rewithdrawal of insulin.

Glucose Monitoring

The 7:00 AM fasting blood glucose level is sufficient for nearly all monitoring of elderly diabetics. Monitoring blood glucose 3–4 hours after each meal, at 11:00 AM, 4:00 PM, and, rarely, 11:00 PM may be helpful for adjusting therapy in some difficult cases. Two-hour postprandial blood sugar levels provide little information about diabetic control. Routine fasting blood sugar monitoring is typically done monthly in asymptomatic, stable patients, but this decision should be individualized. A portable glucometer should be available on every long-term care nursing unit where there are diabetic patients.

References

1. Goldberg AP, Andres R, Bierman EL. Diabetes mellitus in the elderly. In: Hazzard WR, Andres R, Bierman EL, Blass JP (eds). Principles of geriatric medicine and gerontology. New York: McGraw-Hill, 1990:739.
2. Harris M. Epidemiology of diabetes mellitus among the elderly in the United States. Clin Geriatr Med 1990;6:703.
3. Trilling J. Screening for non-insulin-dependent diabetes mellitus in the elderly. Clin Geriatr Med 1990;6:839.
4. Froom J. Glycemic control in elderly people with diabetes. Clin Geriatr Med 1990;6:933.
5. Morley J, Kaiser F. Unique aspects of diabetes mellitus in the elderly. Clin Geriatr Med 1990;6:693.

6. Moller D, Flier J. Insulin resistance—mechanisms, syndromes, and implications. N Engl J Med 1991;325:938.
7. Kaplan N. Two dilemmas of diabetes. Arch Intern Med 1991;151:1270.
8. Laws A, Reaven G. Effect of physical activity on age-related glucose intolerance. Clin Geriatr Med 1990;6:849.
9. Peters A, Davidson M. Insulin plus a sulfonylurea agent for treating Type II diabetes. Ann Intern Med 1991;115:45.
10. Peters A, Davidson M. Use of sulfonylurea agents in older patients. Clin Geriatr Med 1990;6:903.
11. Kitabchi A, Rumbak M. The management of diabetic emergencies. Hosp Pract 1989;129.
12. Wadden T. Long-term glycemic control in patients with Type II diabetes. Arch Intern Med 1991;151:1269.
13. Nathan D. Insulin treatment in the elderly diabetic patient. Clin Geriatr Med 1990;6:923.

13

Prevention and Treatment of Peptic Disease

Philip Gaziano

The prevalence of upper gastrointestinal diseases, which increases with age, accounts for 27% of all hospitalizations of elderly patients and 20% of their deaths (1). Major risk factors for peptic ulcer disease and gastritis are use of nonsteroidal anti-inflammatory drugs (NSAIDs) (2, 3), smoking (2, 4), ethanol consumption, concomitant infection with *Helicobacter pylori,* and changes related to aging, including delayed gastric emptying of liquids (5–7) and achlorhydria (5, 8, 9). Achlorhydria is often accompanied by a decrease in production of protective mucus and prostaglandin E_1, an increase in degradative enzymes such as pepsin, increased gastrin, and a predisposition to *H. pylori* infection.

Diagnosing peptic disease in the elderly may be difficult because dyspeptic symptoms may be attributed to other diseases, and neuropathy from diabetes or other causes may obscure disease presentation. Paradoxically, use of NSAIDs may delay diagnosis by reducing pain from the disease to which they contribute (2).

GASTRIC ULCER

Ninety percent of gastric ulcers occur after the age of 40 years, and account for about one-half of peptic ulcers in patients over 60 years of age and nearly all of those requiring surgery. In patients over 70 years, ulcers occur more proximally on the lesser curvature of the stomach, and are more often associated with decreased acid production, achlorhydria, and gastric cancer. Some proximal ulcers occur in hiatal hernias, which also increase in frequency with age, and have pain referral patterns that resemble cardiac disease. About one-half of hiatal hernia ulcers bleed (10).

Gastric ulcers in older patients tend to be larger, bleed more often (and without prior warning symptoms), and take longer to heal, in part, because of delays in diagnosis and treatment. Of all ulcers in patients over 50 years of age, 10% are greater than 3 cm at presentation, and 10% of these large ulcers are associated with malignancy (2). Barium studies are not as useful as endoscopy in identifying malignancies. Because of the increased association with gastric cancer, which has a high 5-year survival rate after resection, and the association with other gastric pathology including *H. pylori* infections, endoscopy is strongly recommended for most older patients with suspected or known gastric ulcers, rather than a trial of medical management, as might be used in young adults.

Gastric ulcers should be treated with H_2-antagonists (two to four times daily depending on the agents) or proton pump inhibitors for a full 12 weeks (11). Shorter courses and once-daily H_2-antagonist therapy are less effective. Failure to heal an ulcer in 12 weeks, except for large ulcers (>3 cm), usually indicates noncompliance with therapy, concomitant *H. pylori* infection, or malignancy. NSAIDs should be discontinued if possible, but if necessary, may be restarted after ulcer therapy has begun. Gastric ulcers can also be treated with high-dose, frequently administered antacids, but antacid therapy is less effective, relatively expensive, and inconvenient. Omeprazole and misoprostol are probably effective therapy for gastric ulcer, but sucralfate is not.

DUODENAL ULCER

Duodenal ulcers tend to bleed more readily than gastric ulcers, have a higher likelihood of perforation if large, but are less associated with malignancy. Unlike duodenal ulcers in younger patients, excessive acid production is uncommon, perhaps because of the gradual decline in acid output that occurs with aging.

They tend to heal more quickly than gastric ulcers; 8 weeks of therapy with H_2-antagonists is usually adequate. Because of the infrequent association with cancer, empiric treatment without endoscopy or biopsy is reasonable. Maintenance therapy with once-daily H_2-antagonists will reduce the recurrence rate (often asymptomatic) and should be considered in patients over 65 years old with recurrent duodenal ulcer disease.

NSAIDs have a greater effect on the gastric lining than that of the duodenum, but also increase the risk of duodenal ulcers. *H. pylori* infection, thus, should be considered as a factor in recurrent or complicated duodenal ulcers, although the etiological relationship is not as well established as with gastric ulcers or gastritis.

GASTRITIS

Gastritis is more common than duodenal or gastric ulcers, and while it shares with them many risk factors, unlike ulcer disease, advanced age itself is an important independent risk factor for gastritis. Age-related changes in the stomach may be responsible for the observed increased risk: Achlorhydria occurs in 20–50% of patients over 70 years, and age-related increases in gastrin levels delay gastric emptying and increase pepsin production.

Autoimmune gastritis (type A) involves the gastric body and fundus. All type A gastritis patients have parietal cell antibodies, but only one-third develop intrinsic factor antibodies, of which another one-third develop pernicious anemia. Type B gastritis, the most common type in North America, does not have an autoimmune etiology, but is caused by

---

H. pylori, *now believed to be the major cause of Type B gastritis, is a treatable infection . . .*

---

injury from alcohol, smoking, viral illnesses, duodenal reflux, stress, food trauma, and most commonly, NSAID use and *H. pylori* infection.

H. pylori, now believed to be the major cause of Type B gastritis, is a treatable infection that is more common in lower socioeconomic classes and in the elderly (12). Superficial infection without gastritis is present in the great majority of elderly long-term care patients, and predisposes them to the development of gastritis from other gastric injury.

Treatment of gastritis includes reducing acid production with H_2-antagonists or omeprazole, reducing pepsin damage with sucralfate, or protecting the gastric lining with misoprostol, and attempts to eradicate *H. pylori* in appropriate cases.

H. PYLORI INFECTION

H. pylori is a spiral, noninvasive, Gram-negative rod found in the mucous layer of the stomach attached to the surface of mucin-secreting cells (12). The gastric mucous layer apparently protects it from the bactericidal effect of gastric acid and enzymes, lethal to most bacteria. Infection may be diagnosed by antral biopsy, rarely by culture, and by a breath test for carbon-13- or carbon-14-labeled CO_2. Serum *H. pylori* antibodies are nonspecific but may suggest infection. It appears to be spread person to person and is found in most patients in chronic care facilities with up to 75% of those infected having subclinical type B gastritis.

There are several strategies for treating *H. pylori* infection, although no effective single drug therapy has yet been found. One successful triple drug regimen includes 2 weeks of concomitant Pepto-Bismol, 2 tablets q6h; metronidazole, 250 mg q8h; and either tetracycline, 500 mg, or amoxicillin, 500 mg q8h. Failures are common if single- or double-drug therapy or shorter courses are used. Reinfection is common in the chronic care setting and, at present, eradication should be attempted only for recurrent or difficult to treat peptic disease. More effective therapy may, however, make aggressive treatment a reasonable option in the future (13, 14).

THERAPY

Antacids

Bicarbonate, phosphate, or hydroxide salts of calcium, magnesium, and aluminum effectively neutralize gastric acid, but only for about 2 hours after each dose. Sodium salts, such as baking soda, complicate the management of congestive heart failure (CHF), hypertension, or renal disease and should not be used. Sodium is often an impurity found in other antacids as well.

Calcium and magnesium antacids should be avoided in patients with renal failure. Aluminum hydroxide salts, as in Amphojel and AlternaGEL, are the safest in renal failure patients, although aluminum may accumulate and is suspected as a contributing cause of dementia. Antacids, while useful as diagnostic or p.r.n. medications, have largely been replaced by H_2-antagonists (Table 13.1).

H_2-antagonists

Cimetidine, famotidine, and ranitidine are effective at reducing fasting and postprandial gastric acid production. Cimetidine has the shortest half-life and shortest therapeutic effect (4–6 hours after a po dose), and is

Table 13.1.   Peptic Disease Therapy

Agent	Duration of Action (Hours)	DU Dose	GU Dose	Gastritis Dose	Esophageal Reflux Dose	Max Dose
Omeprazole (Prilosec)	24	20–40 mg qhs[a]	20–40 mg qhs[a]	20–40 mg qhs[a]	40 mg qhs[a]	80 mg/day (40 mg b.i.d.)[a]
Ranitidine (Zantac)	12	150 mg b.i.d. 150–300 qhs[a]	150 mg b.i.d.[a]	150 mg b.i.d.[a]	150 mg b.i.d.[a]	150 mg t.i.d.[a]
Famotidine (Pepsid)	8	20–40 mg qhs[a]	20–40 mg qhs[a]	20–40 mg qhs[a]	20–40 mg b.i.d.[a]	80 mg q.i.d.[a]
Cimetidine (Tagamet)	6–8	800 mg qhs[a]	300 mg q.i.d. 800 mg qhs[a]	300 mg q.i.d.[a]	300 mg q.i.d.[a]	800 mg q.i.d.[a]
Sucralfate (Carafate)	6–8		1 g q.i.d.	1 g q.i.d.		1 g q.i.d.
Misoprostal (Cytotec)	6–8		100–200 μg b.i.d. to q.i.d.[a]	100–200 μg b.i.d. to q.i.d.[a]		200 μg q.i.d.[a]
Antacids	2–4	5–30 ml q2–4h	5–30 ml q2–4h	5–30 ml q2–4h	5–30 ml q2–4h	5–30 ml q2–4h

[a]Typical full adult doses. Dosing should be lowered and dosing intervals should be less frequent for the frail elderly and those with impaired hepatic or renal function.

most often given three to four times a day in 300- or 400-mg doses when treating active ulcer disease. It is metabolized in the liver but its half-life is also increased in renal failure. Dosing intervals should be increased in patients with either liver or renal impairment. It is more likely to cause central nervous system (CNS) side effects than the other H_2-antagonists.

Famotidine and ranitidine have longer half-lives with acid suppression for 10–12 hours, allowing them to be used twice daily in acute ulcer disease, and once a day at bedtime for prophylaxis or maintenance therapy. They are excreted renally. The usual oral doses of famotidine are 20 mg b.i.d. or 20–40 mg at bedtime; for ranitidine, the dosages are 150 mg b.i.d. or 150–300 mg at bedtime.

All three are available in parenteral preparations and may be given intramuscularly. Parenteral famotidine and cimetidine doses are the same as for their oral preparations, but the ranitidine dose must be changed to 50 mg 8h when given parenterally. The dosing interval for famotidine and ranitidine should be doubled or tripled in renal failure patients. All three have infrequent but important reversible CNS side effects.

Proton Pump Inhibitors

Omeprazol reduces acid secretion, but by a different mechanism than H_2-antagonists; it also has antibacterial activity against *H. pylori* and may eradicate it when used with amoxicillin. It is most often dosed once a day, gives longer acid suppression than the H_2-antagonists, and is well tolerated, although there is little experience with it in the elderly.

Misoprostol

Misoprostol is a synthetic analog of prostaglandin E_1. It reduces acid secretion slightly and, more importantly, increases mucous and bicarbonate production, thus protecting the gastric lining from acid and pepsin degradation. It is less effective in lowering gastric acid than H_2-antagonists or omeprazole, and is not recommended as initial therapy for peptic disorders.

Disadvantages of misoprostol include the need for frequent dosing (usually four times a day) and abdominal pain and diarrhea in one-fourth of patients. Side effects are less frequent if misoprostol is begun at 100 μg b.i.d. and advanced slowly over 1–2 weeks.

Sucralfate

Sucralfate is a pepsin binder that coats gastric lining defects; it does not reduce acid production, although it may buffer acid to some degree. *Sucralfate* does not interfere with other antacid therapy and has few side effects. Its disadvantage is the need for frequent dosing (usually four times a day) of large tablets that are difficult to swallow. It is less effective for ulcer disease than H_2-antagonists or omeprazolee; it is overused in combination regimens with H_2-antagonists, for which there is rarely need.

Continuous Gastric Feedings and Peptic Disease

Continuous gastric feedings dilute, buffer, and neutralize gastric acid, and effectively treat or prevent peptic disease. Feedings are protective only when given by nasogastric or gastric tubes, and not with jejunal tubes.

References

1. McCarthy D. Smoking and ulcer—time to quit. N Engl J Med 1984;311:726.
2. McCarthy D. Acid peptic disease in the elderly. Clin Geriatr Med 1991;7:231.
3. Cockel R. NSAIDs—Should every prescription carry a government warning? Gut 1987;28:515.
4. Peptic Ulcer Disease. In: The Health Benefits of Smoking Cessation - A Report of the Surgeon General. Rockville, MD: Dept. of Health and Human Services, 1990:429.
5. Francis S. Aging and the stomach. Clin Gastroenterol 1985;14:657.
6. Evans M, Triggs J, Cheung M, et al. Gastric emptying rate in the elderly: implications for drug therapy. J Am Geriatr Soc 1981;29:273.
7. Moore J, Tweedy C, Christian P, Datz F. Effect of age on gastric emptying of liquid and solid meals in men. Dig Dis Sci 1983;28:340.
8. Okada M, Yao T, Fuchigami J. Factors influencing the healing rate of gastric ulcer in hospitalized subjects. Gut 1984:25:881.
9. Tatsuda M, Okuda S. Age related changes in the acid secreting area in patients with duodenal ulcer. *Endoscopy* 1983;15:243.
10. Gilinsky N. Peptic ulcer disease in the elderly. Gastroenterol Clin North Am 1990;19:255.
11. Howden C, Jones D, Peace K, et al. The treatment of gastric ulcer with anti-secretory drugs: relationship of pharmacological effect to healing rates. Dig Dis Sci 1988;33:619.
12. Green L, Graham D. Gastritis in the elderly. Gastroenterol Clin North Am 1990;19:273.
13. Moss S, Calam J. *Helicobacter pylori* and peptic ulcers. the present position. Gut 1992;33:289.
14. Peterson WL. *Helicobacter pylori* and peptic ulcer disease. N Engl J Med 1991;324:1043.

14

Treatment of Chronic Obstructive Pulmonary Disease

Philip Gaziano

Chronic obstructive pulmonary disease (COPD) is predominantly a disease of men, although male predominance has fallen from 6:1 a decade ago to 2.5:1 at the present time, due to increased smoking among women (1). Overall, 14% of men and 8% of women have some form of COPD (2), and prevalence increases with age. Although the three major types of COPD—chronic bronchitis, emphysema, and asthmatic bronchitis—to some degree have distinct pathophysiologies, it is common to encounter features of each type of COPD in the same patient (1–4).

Treatment of COPD must address both the inflammatory and the bronchospastic components of symptomatic obstruction. Up to 40% of older COPD patients have significant bronchospasm, although only a fraction receive bronchodilator therapy (3). Reversible bronchospasm may be detected by a response to bronchodilator therapy during pulmonary function testing, or empirically when therapy improves respiratory function during daily activity. Triggers of bronchospasm include smoke, ozone, and other pollutants, cold weather, changes in humidity or barometric pressure, exercise, dust, molds, possibly foods and food additives, aspirin or NSAIDs, chemical vapors, and infections (4). Therapy includes removing offending triggers and bronchodilation with β-agonist or anticholinergic sympathomimetic agents; patients who develop bronchospasm from predictable irritant exposure, such as cold air or dust, or exercise may benefit from preventive administration of cromolyn sodium or β-agonists before exertion or irritant exposure. The use of anti-inflammatory drugs and antibiotics can reduce bronchial obstruction from inflammation and infection, when present. Table 14.1 gives combined strategies used to treat exacerbations and chronically symptomatic COPD.

Long-term therapy after exacerbations of COPD have subsided must incorporate the prevention of more endothelial damage and irritation

Table 14.1.   Treatment of COPD Exacerbations

Agent	Mild Exacerbations	Moderate Exacerbations	Severe Exacerbations
Albuterol MDI (Proventil, Ventolin)	2 puffs p.r.n. only to 2 t.i.d. and p.r.n.	2 q4h and p.r.n. to 2 puffs as often as needed	> >
Inhaled Corticosteroids (Azmacort MDI)	2 puffs b.i.d. to 2 puffs t.i.d.	4 puffs q.i.d.	
Ipratropium (Atrovent MDI)	2 puffs t.i.d.	2 puffs q.i.d. to 3 puffs q.i.d.	
Albuterol (oral) (Proventil, Ventolin)		2–4 mg at hs to 2–4 mg b.i.d.	4 mg t.i.d.
Prednisone (starting dose/ taper length)		40 mg/day for 8 days	60 mg/day for 12 days to 80 mg/ day for 16 days
Aminophylline (sustained release)			300 mg b.i.d. to 400 mg t.i.d.

from smoking or second-hand smoke, or other inhaled irritants. For patients with severe COPD, there should be an assessment of the need for intermittent or 24-hour oxygen therapy to increase their functional level and, hopefully, to prevent complications of chronic hypoxemia. Physical therapy, occupational therapy, and attention to nutritional status are important to maximize functional status of all older patients disabled by breathlessness.

COPD symptoms may be worsened by non-COPD pulmonary changes associated with aging—decreased mucociliary clearance, decreased compliance of both the chest wall and lungs, some reduction in gas exchange surface area, an increased functional residual capacity, decreased pulmonary vascular regulation, and decreased CO_2 and O_2 sensitivity of brain stem respiratory centers (1, 5, 6). Most presumably age-related deteriorations in respiratory function occur more rapidly in persons with COPD, however. Some of the many concomitant problems that are common in the elderly that may reduce ventilatory function and worsen symptoms of COPD include congestive heart failure (CHF), past thoracic injury or surgery, lung cancer, nonpulmonary infections, and neurological disorders (or drugs) that depress respiratory drive.

THERAPY

Sympathomimetic (β-Agonist) Agents

β-Selective sympathomimetic agents are usually effective as initial treatment of chronically symptomatic and acute exacerbations of COPD: albuterol (Proventil, Ventolin), metaproterenol (Alupent, Metaprel), and terbutaline (Brethine, Bricanyl), all of which are available in metered dose inhalers and oral preparations.

Albuterol and metaproterenol are available in orally dosed liquids and solutions for updraft machines, and terbutaline has a parenteral preparation that may be given subcutaneously. Because albuterol has increased selectively for the bronchial (β_2) receptors, producing less cardiac (β_1) stimulation compared with metaproterenol and terbutaline, it is the initial drug of choice.

Sympathomimetic agents should ordinarily be administered to acutely symptomatic patients by aerosolization through updraft or metered dose inhaler (MDI), which gives high pulmonary tissue levels and reduces their systemic side effects. The major limitations of inhaled dosing for the elderly is their need to understand and cooperate as well as the short duration of activity of the drug. If patients are confused or unable to cooperate, they will probably not receive an adequate dose of drug. Supervised updraft administration is more reliable than MDIs for unreliable or uncooperative patients, but it is also an expensive and labor-intensive method. When done properly, however, MDI is equally effective. The use of "spacers" with MDI eliminates much of the need to concentrate on coordination of inspiration with dose release, and will improve medication delivery for most frail older patients. Mask administration is also possible for acutely ill patients who are unable to cooperate with updraft or MDI.

Oral administration of β-agonists provides a more sustained drug effect, which is particularly useful at night or when the severity of symptoms requires frequent inhaled doses, but at the cost of increased side effects. Theophylline's historic role as a first-line oral bronchodilator has now been replaced by inhaled and p.o. β-agonists, which are safer and provide more specific therapy.

Adverse effects of sympathomimetic agents include anxiety, tremor, tachycardia, insomnia, and nausea.

Theophylline and Aminophylline

It is not clear whether theophylline or aminophylline is beneficial for the treatment of chronically symptomatic or acute exacerbations of COPD. Some studies have shown benefit (7), even when added to β-agonists (8), and others have demonstrated toxicity but no symptomatic benefits (9). There is no doubt, however, that theophylline and aminophylline are particularly hazardous drugs for the elderly (9, 10). Side effects include nausea, diarrhea, agitation, and delirium, potentially fatal cardiac arrhythmias, a reduced seizure threshold, and worsening of Parkinson's disease. Clinically important drug interactions

---

It is not clear whether theophylline or aminophylline is beneficial for the treatment of chronically symptomatic or acute exacerbations of COPD.

---

occur with theophylline; ciprofloxacin (but not ofloxacin) and erythromycin (but not clarithromycin), antibiotics commonly used for respiratory infection, may raise theophylline levels dramatically by inhibition of excretion, resulting in potentially life-threatening toxicity. In addition, acute illness itself slows metabolism, and may result in higher theophylline levels.

In general, β-selective sympathomimetic agents are safer but if theophylline is required, a low-dose sustained-release preparation without a loading dose is preferred (11). It is possible that the standard therapeutic range reported by laboratories is too high for the elderly: Aiming for a lower therapeutic range of 8–15 mg/dl is advisable (12), although life-threatening toxicity in the elderly may be an age-related pharmacodynamic change and is not predictable by drug-level monitoring (10).

Ipratropium and Atropine-like Agents

Ipratropium (Atrovent), administered by updraft or MDI, has anticholinergic activity that gives a bronchodilator effect and also reduces respiratory secretions. It may be used either as initial or sole therapy in chronically symptomatic COPD, or used as adjuvant therapy with sympathomimetics.

Oral preparations of atropine, anisotropine (Valpin), belladonna (e.g., Donnatol), or glycopyrrolate (e.g., Robinul), have little bronchodilatory effect, but have been used to reduce secretions in the respiratory tract. Oral atropine-like therapy provides minimal benefit compared with bronchodilator therapy although a small number of patients with heavy mucous sputum production may be helped. Low-dose tricyclic antidepressants and antihistamines also may provide mild anxiolytic as well as anticholinergic activity without respiratory depression. Side effects of oral atropine-like agents include dry mouth, constipation, urinary retention, drowsiness, and rarely, hypotension. Side effects are rare with ipratropium because of lack of systemic absorption after MDI or updraft administration.

A mucolytic agent, iodinated glycerol (e.g., Organidin), was shown to reduce cough and to assist in clearing sputum in a large controlled study, and may be beneficial in acute exacerbations or chronically symptomatic COPD (13).

Corticosteroids

A subgroup of patients with COPD benefits from the anti-inflammatory effect of corticosteroids. Unfortunately, it is not possible to predict reliably who will respond to corticosteroids, and who will be harmed by their many and often severe adverse effects (14). A therapeutic trial, therefore, is justifiable in patients whose symptoms persist with maximal sympathomimetic therapy.

Inhaled corticosteroids cause fewer systemic effects, and are preferred for initial and long-term therapy. Either form of corticosteroids, however, should be considered primarily as adjunctive treatment for patients already receiving sympathomimetics or ipratropium. Oral therapy should be reserved for acute exacerbations, and should be given as a high-dose short-term regimen that is tapered and discontinued over a few weeks. By any route of administration, including intravenous administration, therapeutic action does not occur for 12–24 hours.

With both inhaled and oral dosing, the most common mistakes are those of undertreatment—underdosing and tapering too rapidly. They are readily absorbed and highly bioavailable, so oral or inhaled administration is preferable to parenteral administration. The major short-term systemic adverse effects are hyperglycemia (or worsening of diabetic control), predisposition to infection, fluid retention, possibly gastric irritation, psychosis and delirium, and muscle weakness. Inhaled corticosteroids also cause oral candidiasis, which may be avoided by having patients rinse their mouth after MDI administration. Long-term systemic use is hazardous, and when chronic corticosteroid therapy is required, frequent inhaled doses by MDI are safer. Long-term therapy causes Cushing's syndrome, osteoporosis, cataracts, skin fragility, reactivation of quiescent tuberculosis, and generally impaired immune function.

It is important to remember to give "stress doses" of corticosteroids to patients receiving long-term therapy who become acutely ill, regardless of the type of acute stress, e.g., infection, injury, stroke, myocardial infarction.

Antibiotics

As is true of many therapies for acute exacerbation of COPD, the efficacy of antibiotic therapy has been questioned for decades. Recent studies have tended to demonstrate benefit from empiric antibiotic therapy, however, even in patients who do not have clear clinical indications of bacterial bronchitis (15).

Antibiotics chosen to treat acute bronchitis complicating COPD in long-term care must cover common Gram-positive and institutionally acquired Gram-negative organisms, such as *H. influenzae*, enterobacteriaceae, or *M. catarrhalis* (Table 14.2) (15). In contrast to community-acquired pneumonia, *S. pneumoniae* is relatively infrequently encountered as a pathogen, especially in elderly residents of long-term care, where, typically, no pathogen can be cultured (about two-thirds of patients), mixed pathogens are cultured (about 10–15%),

Table 14.2. Broad-spectrum Oral Empiric Antibiotic Therapy for Acute Exacerbation of COPD[a]

Co-trimoxazole (Bactrim, Septra, generic), 1 DS tablet b.i.d.
Ofloxacin (Floxin), 400 mg b.i.d.
Amoxicillin/clavulanate (Augmentin), 500 mg t.i.d.
Cefixime (Suprax), 400 mg qday
Clarithromycin (Biaxin), 500 mg b.i.d.

[a]Includes activity against *S. pneumoniae, m. catarrhalis, h. influenzae,* and enterobacteriacae.

or a Gram-negative bacillus is cultured about 15–25% (16). It is possible, moreover, that atypical organisms such as *Chlamydia* or *Mycoplasma* species which are not routinely culturable and are not usually associated with productive cough, may play a role as coinfecting agents (12). Sputum cultures are, therefore, not cost-effective, and are more likely to misguide than to guide therapy.

Traditionally employed antibiotics, such as amoxicillin, tetracycline, or the first- and second-generation oral cephalosporins, such as cephalexin or cefaclor, have limited Gram-negative coverage and should not be used for empiric therapy of serious infections (see Chapter 3). Co-trimoxazole and the new quinolones, such as ofloxacin (17), offer better activity against both typical and atypical respiratory pathogens, and are well tolerated. Parenteral antibiotics are rarely necessary, unless patients cannot take oral therapy.

Metered-dose Inhalers (MDI)

MDI administration conveniently delivers pulmonary medications to respiratory tissues with little systemic absorption of most medications, thereby greatly reducing toxicity. In addition, MDI administration offers the theoretical advantage of delivering greater concentrations of drug to pulmonary tissues than could be achieved or tolerated by parenteral administration.

There is, however, a serious risk of unrecognized undertreatment of elderly patients receiving MDI therapy in long-term care. Proper use of MDIs requires the coordination of deep inhalation, closing of nares, and triggering of the medication release—any of which may be difficult for weak, confused, or ill elderly patients. Even if long-term care nursing staff are aware of the need to instruct, to monitor, and to supervise MDI administration, oral or parenteral therapy may be safer for acutely ill patients. Reliability of dose delivery in frail or acutely ill elderly patients will be improved by the use of spacers on MDIs.

References

1. Webster JR. Unique aspects of respiratory disease in the aged. Geriatrics 1991;431.
2. Higgins M. Epidemiology of COPD: state of the art. Chest 1984;85:3S.
3. Banerjee DK. Underdiagnosis of asthma in the elderly. Br J Dis Chest 1987;81:23.
4. Rumbak MJ. New concepts in treatment of chronic persistent asthma using a stepwise protocol to control inflammation. Postgrad Med 1991;90:81.
5. Mahler D. Chronic obstructive pulmonary disease. Clin Geriatr Med 1986;2:285.
6. Mahler D. The aging lung. Geriatr Clin North Am 1986;2:215.
7. Filuk RB, Easton PA, Anthonisen NR. Responses to large doses of salbutamol and theophylline in patients with chronic obstructive pulmonary disease. Am Rev Respir Dis 1985;132:871.
8. Wrenn K, Slovis CM, Murphy F, Greenberg RS. Aminophylline therapy for acute bronchospastic disease in the emergency room. Ann Intern Med 1991;115:241.
9. Rice KL, Leatherman JW, Duane PG, et al. Aminophylline for acute exacerbations of chronic obstructive pulmonary disease. A controlled trial. Ann Intern Med 1987;107:305.
10. Shannon M, Lovejoy FH. The influence of age vs. peak serum concentration of life-threatening events after chronic theophylline intoxication. Arch Intern Med 1990;150:2045.
11. Poe R. Theophylline in asthma and COPD: changing perspectives and controversies. Geriatrics 1991;46:55.
12. Nicotra MB, Waldrop D, Stocks JM. Therapy for acute exacerbations of chronic bronchitis. Geriatr Infect Dis 1992;2:1.
13. Petty TL. The national mucolytic study: results of a randomized, double-blind, placebo-controlled study of iodinated glycerol in chronic obstructive bronchitis. Chest 1990;97:75.
14. Hudson LD, Monti CM. Rationale and use of corticosteroids in chronic obstructive pulmonary disease. Med Clin North Am 1990;74:661.
15. Anthonisen NR, Manfreda J, Warren CPW, et al. Antibiotic therapy in exacerbations of chronic obstructive pulmonary disease. Ann Intern Med 1987;106:196.
16. Yoshikawa TT. Treatment of nursing home-acquired pneumonia. J Am Geriatr Soc 1991;39:1040.
17. Stocks JM, Wallace RL, Griffith DE, et al. Ofloxacin in community-acquired lower respiratory infections. A comparison with amoxicillin or erythromycin. Am J Med 1989;87:52S.

15

Evaluating Drug Therapy: Principles and Practices for Long-term Care Providers

Edward G. Tessier

Awareness of the need to reduce so-called polypharmacy in the elderly has been growing over the past two decades (1–9) and is reflected in new regulatory standards (10, 11). The Omnibus Budget Reconciliation Act of 1987, first implemented in October of 1990 (10) and revised in September of 1991 for April 1992 implementation (11) states that "each resident's drug regimen must be free from unnecessary drugs." An 'unnecessary drug' is broadly defined for the purposes of this regulation as a drug that is used "in excessive dose, for excessive duration, without adequate monitoring, without adequate indications for its use, or in the presence of adverse consequences which indicate the dose should be reduced or discontinued . . ." Specific criteria for antipsychotic drug use and proposed criteria for benzodiazepine use are also delineated in the regulation or in related interpretative guidelines (See Chapter 7; Sedative Hypnotics and Antipsychotics). While the physician is not directly penalized for violation, failure to adhere to these regulations may jeopardize a facility's Medicare and Medicaid funding.

Health care providers may justly complain that such regulatory approaches are coercive rather than helpful, but few could argue against the intent of the regulations. If the new regulatory standards result in adoption of a systematic approach in the evaluation of drug therapy as a cooperative effort by the physician, consulting pharmacist, nursing staff, and the facility, it will have been a worthwhile strategy that focuses both on the drug regimen of the individual patient and overall drug use in the facility.

PATIENT-SPECIFIC EVALUATION OF DRUG THERAPY

Drug Regimen Review

The drug regimen review (DRR) is intended to serve as the primary systematic means to evaluate drug therapy in most long-term care settings. Medicare and Medicaid requirements mandate that "the drug regimen of each resident must be reviewed at least once a month by a licensed pharmacist." Furthermore, the pharmacist "must report any irregularities to the attending physician and the director of nursing, and these reports must be acted upon" (9). The implication is that identification of drug therapy problems is not sufficient—an attempt by the physician must be made to act on recommendations made in the drug regimen review or to document why those recommendations are not being followed.

Requirements for DRR in Intermediate Care Facilities for the Mentally Retarded (ICF/MR) fall under different regulations (12), requiring the pharmacist to perform the DRR on a quarterly basis and to provide input to the interdisciplinary team. In ICF/MR settings, the pharmacist must also participate in the development, implementation, and review of each client's individual program plan, specifically as it relates to drug therapy used to control maladaptive behaviors.

The drug regimen review should include at least an evaluation of the appropriateness of and response to each patient's drug therapy. The Health Care Financing Administration has adopted indicators (objectively measured standards signifying patterns of performance) for state agency surveyors to assess the quality of DRRs (Appendix 15.1) (13). Application of the federal indicators to the nursing home DRR has been associated with improved adherence to stop-order policies and reduced continuous use of p.r.n. medications, but has not been associated with reduced overall medication use (14). Automated systems that link these indicators with computer-based patient medication profiles are available and serve as the framework for the DRR in many settings (15). Such integrated systems can improve the efficiency of the pharmacist conducting the DRR by flagging duplicate medication use, potential drug interactions, or doses outside a predetermined range; they can also identify indications for periodic laboratory monitoring for particular drugs. Their utility, however, is limited: the significance of identified interactions, assessment of patient response to therapy, or appropriateness of alternative therapeutic options requires clinician judgment.

Unfortunately, the effectiveness of currently mandated DRRs in improving medication use in long-term care settings has been recently questioned, based upon a review of published studies of interventions to improve medication use in nursing home settings (5). Only time-consuming face-to-face educational interventions, including an educational component for nursing staff, reliably improves utilization of medication use.

Thus, merely performing a DRR by following the HCFA indicators does not necessarily result in reduced medication use or improved clinical outcomes. A commitment to judicious drug use by the physician, pharmacist, nurse, and facility in conjunction with a broader DRR that addresses the patient's response to drug and nondrug interventions is necessary to optimize therapy. The American Society of Consultant Pharmacists has incorporated these broader considerations into their guidelines for assessing quality DRRs. An overview of their guidelines is presented in Appendix 15.2. An example of a problem-oriented DRR is presented in Figure 15.1.

Long-term Care Facility XYZ
Drug Regimen Review

Patient Name: __Jane Doe__ Age: __83__
Room number: __205A__ Date: __12/5/91__
Physician: __Ellen Jones__

1. *Congestive Heart Failure/Hypertension:*

Current medications: Digoxin 0.125 mg po qd
Furosemide 40 mg po qd (increased from 20 mg po qod on 11/1/91)
Captopril 12.5 mg po tid (started 11/4/91)

Improvement in respiratory symptoms and petal edema over past 3 weeks per nursing staff. 11/10–12/4: mean BP = 142 ± 12/88 ± 7 n = 45; Apical pulses range 70–85.

Most recent electrolytes on 9/12/91:

138	99	Creatinine 1.1
-----	-----	Est CrCl (Cockcroft-Gault method):
3.5	26	29 ml/min

Last digoxin level 9/4/91 WNL at 1.4 µg/L (Est CrCl at time about 35 ml/min.) No evidence of digoxin toxicity at present.

Recommendation: Would recommend obtaining follow-up electrolytes given increase in furosemide dose, and initiation of Captopril over the past month.

Figure 15.1. Example of drug regimen review.

2. *Dementia/Agitated Behavior:*

Current medications: Thioridazine 50 mg po qd at hs.
(Digoxin 0.125 mg po qd)
(Triazolam 0.25 mg po hs prn—started 8/6/91;
used approx 5–7× per week)

Abnormal Involuntary Movement Scale evaluation performed on 11/15/91 by RPh and RN and revealed no significant involuntary movements. No obvious EPS noted on observation at that time.

Alert on observation today at 10AM. Nursing staff note that agitated behavior includes occasional striking out at staff, yelling, and crying out. Agitated behavior predates use of digoxin/triazolam therapy, although nursing staff note subjective increase in confusion since initiation of triazolam use. While nursing staff note that agitated behavior interferes with staff's ability to provide care, it is unclear if present thioridazine therapy is effective in improving symptoms of agitated behavior.

Recommendation:

a. Consider discontinuation of triazolam in light of suggestion that exacerbation of confusion and agitated behavior coincides with use of the drug (see Insomnia below).

b. Nursing staff, facility staff, and clinical pharmacist establish a means to identify and track the frequency and intensity of agitated behaviors consistent with HCFA regulations and current Drug Use Evaluation for antipsychotics.

c. Nursing and facility staff review options to alter environment and staff response to agitated behaviors.

d. Once data collection and environmental alterations are in place, would consider a reduction in thioridazine dosage in evaluating the effectiveness of antipsychotic therapy if clinically appropriate.

3. *Insomnia:*

Current medication: Triazolam 0.25 mg po hs prn. (Used approximately 5–7x per week since 8/6/91.)

Nursing staff note that patient often awake early in the morning (? early morning insomnia related to chronic triazolam use.) Presently recommended geriatric dosage typically 0.125 mg.

Recommendation: Given increase in agitation and early morning insomnia, would recommend reducing dosage of triazolam to 0.125 mg qhs for 1 week then D/C. Alternately, short-term use of a longer-acting agent (e. g., Temazepam 15 mg po hs × 1 week, then 15 mg po qohs × 1 week, then D/C) may reduce withdrawal symptoms.

Medications reviewed. Recommendations as above.

John Smith, R.Ph.

Figure 15.1.   *Continued.*

Adverse Drug Reaction Monitoring

Monitoring for adverse drug reactions is part of a good DRR. Monitoring for specific adverse reactions (i.e., movement disorders secondary to antipsychotic medication) requires a special effort beyond that of a record-based DRR.

FACILITY-WIDE DRUG EVALUATION

Drug Use Evaluation

Criteria-based evaluation of specific drug use has been a standard of practice in acute care hospitals for a number of years. Drug use evaluation (DUE) is required by the Joint Commission of Accreditation of Healthcare Organizations (JCAHO) in both acute and long-term care settings. Drug use evaluation is a medical staff requirement defined by the JCAHO as a "criteria based, ongoing, planned, and systematic process designed to continuously improve the appropriate and effective

---

Problem-prone, frequently used drugs are ideal candidates for DUE studies, . . . antipsychotic agents, anticonvulsants, analgesics, sedative hypnotics, or digoxin.

---

use of drugs" (16). Drug use evaluations can complement the DRR (17) and can be integrated into the quality assessment activities of the long-term care setting (18). A DUE should be conducted on a prospective or concurrent basis, and the results should directly influence patient care. Problem-prone, frequently used drugs are ideal candidates for DUE studies, and, in long-term care settings, may include antipsychotic agents, anticonvulsants, analgesics, sedative hypnotics, or digoxin. DUE can be simple or complex, and varies depending on the nature of the drug, the facility, and the resources available. Two examples of criteria for DUE are presented; Figure 15.2 illustrates a simple DUE for digoxin and Figure 15.3 shows a more complex DUE for antipsychotics that incorporates HCFA requirements regarding indication for antipsychotic use (See Chapter 7; Sedative Hypnotics and Antipsychotics).

Long-term Care Facility XYZ   Patient Name: ___Jane Doe___
Drug Use Evaluation   Room Number: _205A_ Date: __12/5/91__
DIGOXIN   Physician: _____Ellen Jones_____

INDICATION:

Y   N   NA
X   __ __   1. Signs or symptoms of heart failure within the past 2 years?
__ X   __   2. Past electrocardiogram showing:
                    ____ Atrial Fibrillation
                    ____ Atrial Flutter
                    ____ Paroxysmal Atrial Tachycardia?

DOSING:

Y   N   NA
X   __ __   1. Dose range for maintenance dosage 0.125 mg qod to 0.25 mg qd, or
                level obtained?

MANAGEMENT:

Y   N   NA
__ __ X   1. Digoxin level ordered if evidence of digitalis toxicity (nausea, vomiting,
               and/or diarrhea)?
__ X   __   2. If patient on concurrent diuretic, has serum potassium been ordered
               within 30 days of initiating diuretic and every 6 months thereafter?
X   __ __   3. Pulse rate obtained daily during first month of therapy and at least
               weekly thereafter?

Figure 15.2. Example of drug use evaluation—digoxin.

Establishing a DUE program requires a commitment of the medical staff, nursing staff, and the consultant pharmacist to delineate responsibility, identify appropriate drugs to study, establish criteria for appropriate use, implement the study, review the results, and correct patient-specific and facility-wide problem issues, if necessary. The scope of the DUE may be broadened to look at quality-of-life issues; activity staff, for example, may be particularly helpful as objective, impartial observers of daytime sedation related to sedative-hypnotic use.

Adverse Drug Reaction Reporting

An ongoing mechanism of reporting adverse drug reactions is another requirement of the JCAHO for both acute and long-term care settings. To be effective, this requires significant nursing staff involvement in the

Long-term Care Facility XYZ
Drug Use Evaluation
ANTIPSYCHOTICS

Patient Name: __Jane Doe__
Room Number: _205B_ Date: _12/5/91_
Physician: ____Ellen Jones____

INCLUDES: Amoxapine, chlorpromazine, fluphenazine, haloperidol, loxapine, mesoridazine, molindone, perphenazine, pimoxide, thioridazine, trifluoperazine, triflupromazine, thiothixene.

INDICATION:
Y   N   NA

__ __ _X_ 1. Clinical record documents that the patient has one or more of the following:

—Schizophrenia	—Schizo-affective	—Delusional disorder
—Psychotic Mood	disorder	—Brief reactive
Disorder (including	—Acute psychotic	—Atypical psychosis
mania or depres-	episodes	—Huntington's disease
sion with psychotic	—Schizophreniform	
features)	disorder	
	—Tourette's disorder	

AND/OR

__ _X_ __ 2. Organic mental syndromes (including dementia) with associated psychotic and/or agitated features as defined by:

—specific behaviors that are quantitatively (number of episodes) and objectively (e. g., biting, kicking, scratching) documented, which cause the patient to:
  • present danger to him/herself
  • present danger to others
  • actually interfere with staff's ability to provide care.
—psychotic symptoms (hallucinations, paranoia, delusions) not exhibited as specific behaviors listed in "1" above, but which cause the patient frightful distress.

AND/OR

__ __ _X_ 3. Short-term (7 days) symptomatic treatment of hiccups, nausea, vomiting, or pruritis in nonterminal patient.

AND/OR

__ __ _X_ 4. Not used if one or more of the following is/are the only indication:

—Simple pacing	—Wandering	—Poor self-care
—Restlessness	—Impaired memory	—Crying out, yelling,
—Anxiety	—Depression	screaming
—Unsociability	—Fidgeting	—Insomnia
—Nervousness	—Uncooperativeness	—Indifference to
		surroundings

Figure 15.3. Example of drug use evaluation—antipsychotics.

MANAGEMENT:

Y	N	NA	
X	__	__	1. Patient is NOT concomitantly receiving a second antipsychotic agent.
X	__	__	2. Patient is NOT experiencing:

       —Urinary retention   —Orthostatic hypotension
       —Marked sedation after   —Functionally limiting
         1 week   extrapyramidal symptoms.

| | | X | 3. Rationale for antiparkinsonian agent is specified when originally ordered and re-evaluated 60 days after initially instituted. |
| X | __ | __ | 4. AIMS evaluation conducted on quarterly basis and results forwarded to physician. |

Figure 15.3.   *Continued.*

identification and reporting of adverse reactions. Trends in reporting may indicate that a change in policy or restricted use of a particular drug is necessary. Significant or unusual adverse drug reactions should be reported to the FDA; such reports will ultimately add to understanding of how this elderly population responds to drug therapy.

Other Quality Assurance Reports

Medication error reports or safety reports may reveal facility-wide trends requiring changes in policy, procedure, or patterns of care provision. For example, an increase in falls may be noted in patients who are receiving overly aggressive antihypertensive therapy or who are experiencing orthostatic hypotension related to antidepressant therapy. Changes in care patterns (e.g., obtaining orthostatic blood pressures, notifying the attending physician of such changes, adjusting medication appropriately, and training staff on ways to reduce risks of falls in these patients) can ultimately reduce significant risks in this frail population.

INTEGRATING FACILITY-WIDE DRUG EVALUATION WITH THE DRUG REGIMEN REVIEW

The DRR serves as the basic mechanism to evaluate drug therapy on a patient-specific, ongoing basis. The DRR can serve as an important information source during implementation of the DUE or other quality assessment reviews. Information from other reports can also improve the comprehensiveness of the DRR (Fig. 15.4). The DUE serves as the

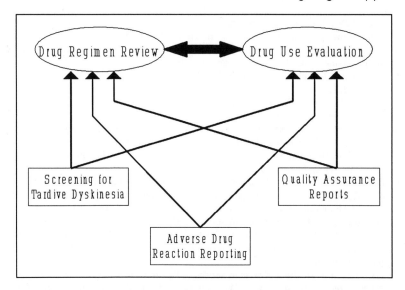

Figure 15.4. Integrating facility-wide drug use evaluation with patient-specific drug regimen review.

basis to review patterns of facility-wide drug use, and to measure those patterns against predetermined criteria established by the medical staff. Integration of patient-specific DUE results into the DRR often leads to improved drug use. Similarly, adverse drug reaction reporting should lead to a re-evaluation of the drug regimen of each patient affected. Medication error or omission reports may highlight a patient-specific compliance problem that should be addressed in the DRR. In addition, trends in adverse drug reactions may prompt a new DUE to help identify means to reduce problems with a particular drug.

References

1. Kalchthaler T, Coccaro E, Lichtiger S. Incidence of polypharmacy in a long-term care facility. J Am Geriatr Soc 1977;25:308.
2. Segal JL, Thompson JF, Floyd RA. Drug utilization and prescribing patterns in a skilled nursing facility: the need for a rational approach to therapeutics. J Am Geriatr Soc 1979;27:117.
3. Roberts PA. Extent of medication use in U.S. long-term-care facilities. Am J Hosp Pharm 1988;45:93.

4. Cooper JW, Bagwell CG. Contribution of the consultant pharmacist to rational drug usage in the long-term care facility. J Am Geriatr Soc 1978;26:513.

5. Gurwitz JH, Soumerai SB, Avorn J. Improving medication prescribing and utilization in the nursing home. J Am Geriatr Soc 1990;38:542.

6. Stewart RB. Polypharmacy in the elderly: a fait accompli? DICP Ann Pharmacother 1990;24:321.

7. Kroenke K, Pinholt EM. Reducing polypharmacy in the elderly—a controlled trial of physician feedback. J Am Geriatr Soc 1990;38:31.

8. Stewart RB, Yedinak KC, Ware MR. Polypharmacy in psychiatry: three case studies and methods of prevention. DICP Ann Pharmacother 1992;26:529.

9. Laucka PV, Hoffman NB. Decreasing medication use in a nursing-home patient-care unit. Am J Hosp Pharm 1992;49:96.

10. Department of Health and Human Services—Health Care Financing Administration 42CFR, part 405, et al. Medicare and Medicaid; requirements for long-term care facilities; final rule with request for comments. Fed Reg 1989;54:ss483.25;5366.

11. Department of Health and Human Services—Health Care Financing Administration 42CFR, parts 431, et al. Medicare and Medicaid; requirements for long-term care facilities and nurse aide training and competency evaluation programs; final rules. Fed Reg 1991;56:48825.

12. Department of Health and Human Services—Health Care Financing Administration 42CFR, parts 431, 435, 440, 442, and 443. Medicaid program; conditions for intermediate care facilities for the mentally retarded; final rules. Fed Reg 1988;53:20447.

13. Indicators for surveyor assessment of the performance of drug regimen reviews. State operations manual, provider certification; Department of Health and Human Services—Health Care Financing Administration. Transmittal No. 242, Appendix N, part 2. September 1990.

14. Shannon RC, DeMuth JE. Application of federal indicators in nursing-home drug-regimen review. Am J Hosp Pharm 1984;41:912.

15. Consultant software—software for consultant pharmacists servicing long-term care and institutional facilities. ComputerTalk 1991;11:80. (ComputerTalk, 1750 Walton Rd, Blue Bell, PA 19422).

16. 1991 Joint Commission Accreditation Manual for Hospitals. Oakbrook Terrace, IL: Joint Commission on Accreditation of Healthcare Organizations, 1991.

17. Hernandez P, Davidson HE, Bauwens SF, Chamberlain TM. Drug use evaluation, part 1: concepts and methods for evaluating the use of drugs in organized health care environments. Consult Pharm 1991;6:643.

18. Feinberg JL. Meeting the mandate for quality assurance through drug use evaluation. Consult Pharm 1991;6:611.

Appendix 15.1. Surveyor Procedures for Pharmaceutical Service Requirements in Long-Term Care Facilities[a]

INDICATORS FOR SURVEYOR ASSESSMENT OF THE PERFORMANCE OF DRUG REGIMEN REVIEW

PART ONE

Indicators for Surveyor Assessment of the Performance of Drug Regimen Reviews

Skilled Nursing Facilities (SNFs) and Intermediate Care Facilities (ICFs) must review the patient's drug regimen at least monthly (42 CFR 405.1127 (a) and 42 CFR 442.336 (a)). In intermediate care facilities for the mentally retarded (ICFs/MR) such reviews must be performed on a regular basis, at least quarterly (42 CFR 483.460 (j) (1)). The reviews must be performed by a pharmacist. Information collected (e.g., drug administration records, physician orders, laboratory reports) is analyzed to determine whether there are any potential problems with the patient's drug therapy, and whether such drug therapy is achieving the stated objectives established by the physician for that patient. If there are potential problems, or if stated objectives are apparently not being achieved, the pharmacist must notify the attending physician.

I. PROPER USE OF INDICATORS

The word indicator describes what you discern as patterns of performance by the pharmacist in the conduct of the required drug regimen reviews. Most of these indicators, taken individually, could not lead to a conclusive finding of compliance or noncompliance with the drug regimen review requirements. However, together with the compliance history of the facility, they could represent reasonable evidence whether the pharmacist is adequately performing drug regimen reviews. If there is a high degree of deviation from these

---

[a]Adapted and reprinted with permission from "Guidelines—Assessing the Quality of Drug Regimen Review in Long-term Care Facilities." Copyright © 1989, American Society of Consultant Pharmacists, Inc.

indicators, *good* reasons for the deviation must be evident from the patient's record. They may often be learned from the pharmacist and, for this reason, it is recommended that the pharmacist be present during the survey of the drug regimen review requirement.

When conducting surveys of SNFs participating in the Medicare program, for the survey to be considered valid, evaluate the pharmacy condition of participation by referring to these indicators. Under the Medicaid program, States have the choices of using these indicators or, alternatively, HCFA accepts other survey criteria developed by the State if it establishes that its criteria are, at a minimum, equal to these indicators in terms of their reliability and objectivity.

II. INDICATORS FOR ASSESSING DRUG REGIMEN REVIEWS

A. Reviews Performed Versus Average Census

Compare the number of drug regimen reviews performed to the average census of the facility. If the average census is 100, the number of reviews that would have been performed *per month* would be about 100. However, this simple indicator is not absolute. Allow tolerances. For example, the pharmacist may have reviewed only 50 percent of the patients in a particular month, but the other 50 percent are scheduled for review the day after the survey. If the number of reviews falls significantly short of the patient census over a number of months, a noncompliance finding is in order.

In ICFs/MR, reviews need be performed only on a quarterly basis. Thus, modify this indicator in the ICF/MR to state that all patients are reviewed quarterly rather than monthly.

B. Reviews Should Be Performed in the Facility

A pharmacist reviewer cannot be *required* to perform reviews in the facility. The regulations do not state where the reviews must be performed. However, in order to perform acceptable reviews, the facility's reviewer must be examining data sources such as the patient's drug administration record, physician orders, nursing notes, and laboratory reports. For all practical purposes these data sources are only located in the facility. Thus, to adequately perform reviews, the pharmacist should conduct them in the facility.

C. Average Prescription Utilization

In 1974, the average prescription utilization per SNF patient was approximately 6.1. The current average is probably unchanged. As a general rule, one could question the adequacy of drug reviews if the facility's average prescription utilization were about 6 per patient. There are qualifications to this indicator:

- The 6.1 average is a national average. Regional and State variations can be significantly different. The average in the State may be more meaningful. The Medicaid Management information System, if one is available, can assist in supplying this information.
- The nature of the patient population (e.g., a high number of patients with multiple chronic diseases) may indicate a higher utilization.
- The assumption that drug regimen reviews reduce utilization may not be true. A drug regimen review may result in additional drug utilization.
- The pharmacist may be performing good reviews and recommending that drugs be discontinued, but the physician may not agree. Your analysis of the *trend* in prescription utilization is critical. The pharmacist may be changing attitudes about drug therapy, and a slow improvement may be evolving. Thus, if the average is higher than 6, but the trend is toward reduction, the pharmacist may be adequately performing drug reviews.
- In an ICF/MR the drug utilization is usually significantly lower (approximately 3 per patient per month). ICF's drug utilization is usually comparable to SNFs.

In order to estimate the average prescription utilization, examine a sufficient number of charts to establish a pattern. It is not necessary to calculate an exact average. In determining the average, include all legend and over-the-counter (OTC) drugs.

Count as one prescription any drug order, including as needed

(PRN) orders, if *one* dose has been administered in the last 30 days. If a drug has been ordered but not administered in the last 30 days, do not count it in the average. Count combination drugs (e. g., aspirin and codeine) as one prescription.

D. Excessive Reviews on the Same Date

The ability of a pharmacist to review patient records is finite. Question the adequacy of review if more than 100 patients have been reviewed on the same day by the same reviewer.

E. Apparent Irregularities (Potential Drug Therapy Problems)

Subsection E.2. lists drug therapy circumstances which *may* constitute drug irregularities (potential drug therapy problems). The pharmacist should address them every time they are encountered. Initially learn five to ten of them and use them in your surveys. Learn an additional five to ten more, and so forth, until all are learned.

1. RULES FOR APPLYING APPARENT IRREGULARITIES

- The pharmacist conducting reviews is responsible for identifying apparent authority of the need to correct the potential problem.
- You are responsible for determining whether such *identification* and *notification* has taken place. Do not go beyond determining if *identification* and *notification* has occurred. *It is not necessary to ascertain the disposition of the recommendation made. Inquiry into the specific treatment or outcome could be construed as Federal Interference with the practice of medicine, which is prohibited by Section 1801 of the Social Security Act.*
- A record of drug regimen reviews must be maintained in the facility to demonstrate that such reviews have been performed. This record may or may not be a part of the patient's medical record depending upon the facility's policy. Each patient must be identified, and documentation of one of the following circumstances must exist:

— If no potential problems were found, the pharmacist reviewer must have included a signed and dated statement to this effect in the drug regimen review record.

— If a potential problem was found and the pharmacist reviewer deemed it *not* significant, he or she must have included a signed and dated statement in the record which describes the situation.

— If a potential significant problem was found, the pharmacist reviewer must have included a signed and dated statement in the record describing the situation and indicating that this information was communicated to an individual with authority to correct it, usually the attending physician.

— The pharmacist reviewer need not have documented the identification and notification every month (or quarter in ICFs/MR) even if the apparent irregularity continues, if it has been deemed insignificant by the pharmacist reviewer, or it has been deemed significant, but the recommendation has been rejected by the individual having authority to correct it.

Under these circumstances, the facility's reviewer may document that he or she has identified an apparent irregularity and notified a person having authority to correct the potential problem on an *annual* basis. This documentation should appear in whatever record the facility uses for documenting drug regimen reviews.

2. LIST OF APPARENT IRREGULARITIES

These drug therapy circumstances *may* constitute drug irregularities (potential drug therapy problems).

NOTE: Generic names are noted only when they are in common usage and are designated by lower case type.

• Multiple orders of the same drug for the same patient by the same route of administration (e.g., the same chemical entity by different brand names);

• Drugs administered in disregard of established stop order policies;

- As needed (PRN) drug orders administered as directed every day for more than 30 days;
- Patients receiving three or more laxatives *concurrently*. Sequential use need not be questioned. Examples of commonly used laxatives are:

Agoral (mineral oil)	glycerin suppositories
Cascara Sagrada (cascara extract)	Haley's M.O.
	Konsyl (psyllium hydrophilic mucilloid)
Chronulac (lactulose)	
Colace (docusate sodium)	Metamucil (psyllium)
Dialose(docusate potassium)	milk of magnesia (MOM)
Dorbantyl (docusate sodium)	(magnesium hydroxide)
Doxinate	Modane Bulk (danthron)
Dulcolax (bisacodyl)	Modane Soft (docusate sodium)
Effer-Syllium (psyllium hydrocolloid)	Neoloid (castor oil)
Fleet Enema (Sodium phosphate/sodium biphosphate)	Peri-Colace (casanthranol)
	Senokot (senna extract)
	Surfak (docusate calcium)

- Use of antipsychotics or antidepressants for fewer than three days. (Exception: Compazine used as an antinauseant).
- *Continuous* use of the following hypnotic (sleep induction) drugs for more than 30 days.

	Usual Maximum Single Dosage Age 65 & Over	Usual Maximum Single Dosage
Amytal	150 mg	300 mg
Butisol (butabarbital)	100 mg	200 mg
Dalmane (flurazepam hydrochloride)	15 mg	30 mg
Doriden	500 mg	1000 mg
Halcion (triazolam)	0.25 mg	0.5 mg
Nembutal (pentobarbital)	100 mg	200 mg
Noctec (chloral hydrate)	750 mg	1500 mg
Noludar (methyprylon)	200 mg	400 mg

Placidyl (ethchlorvynol)	500 mg	1000 mg
Restoril (temazepam)	15 mg	30 mg
Seconal (secobarbital)	100 mg	200 mg

- Use of two or more hypnotic drugs listed above at the same time, or administered in excess of the listed maximum doses:
- Use of two or more of the following antipsychotic drugs at the same time.

	Usual Maximum Daily Antipsychotic Dosage for Ages 65 & Over	Usual Maximum Daily Antipsychotic Dosage
Haldol (haloperidol)	50 mg	100 mg
Loxitane (loxapine)	125 mg	250 mg
Mellaril (thioridazine)	400 mg	800 mg
Moban, Lidone (molindone hydrochloride)	112 mg	225 mg
Navane (thiothixene)	30 mg	60 mg
Proketazine	200 mg	400 mg
Prolixin (fluphenazine)	20 mg	40 mg
Quide	80 mg	160 mg
Repoise	80 mg	160 mg
Serentil (mesoridazine)	250 mg	500 mg
Stelazine (trifluoperazine hydrochloride)	40 mg	80 mg
Taractan (chlorprothixene)	800 mg	1600 mg
Thorazine (chlorpromazine)	800 mg	1600 mg
Tindal	150 mg	300 mg
Trilafon (perphenazine)	32 mg	64 mg
Vesprin	100 mg	200 mg

- Use of the antipsychotic drugs listed in excess of their listed daily dosage maximums;
- Use of a listed antipsychotic drug unless the clinical record documents that one of the following specific conditions exists:

(1) Schizophrenia
(2) Schizo-affective disorder
(3) Delusional disorder
(4) Psychotic mood disorders (including mania and depression with psychotic features)
(5) Acute psychotic episodes
(6) Brief reactive psychosis
(7) Schizophreniform disorder
(8) Atypical psychosis
(9) Tourette's disorder
(10) Huntington's disease
(11) Organic mental syndromes (including dementia) with associated psychotic and/or agitated features as defined by:
   (a) Specific behaviors (e.g., biting, kicking, scratching) which are quantitatively (e.g., number of episodes) documented by the facility and which cause the resident to:
      —Present a danger to themselves
      —Present a danger to others (including staff) or
      —Actually interfere with staff's ability to provide care, or
   (b) *Continuous* crying out, screaming, yelling, or pacing if these specific behaviors cause an *impairment in functional capacity* and if they are quantitatively (e.g., periods of time) documented by the facility, or
   (c) Psychotic symptoms (hallucinations, paranoia, delusions) not exhibited as specific behaviors listed in "a" and "b" above if these behaviors cause an *impairment in functional capacity*.
(12) Short-term (7 days) symptomatic treatment of hiccups, nausea, vomiting, or pruritus.
- Use of the antipsychotic drugs in the absence of gradual dose reduction attempted every six months after therapy began. Gradual dose reductions are not necessary if within the last six months the resident has had a gradual dose reduction and

the dose has been reduced to the lowest possible dose to control symptoms.

- Use of a listed antipsychotic drug when one or more of the following behaviors is the only indication for use:
  (1) Wandering
  (2) Poor self-care
  (3) Restlessness
  (4) Impaired memory
  (5) Anxiety
  (6) Depression
  (7) Insomnia
  (8) Unsociability
  (9) Indifference to surroundings
  (10) Fidgeting
  (11) Nervousness
  (12) Uncooperativeness
  (13) Unspecified agitation
- The use of a p.r.n. antipsychotic drug more than five times in any 7-day period without a review of the resident's condition by a physician.
- Use of the following anxiolytic drugs when their dosages exceed the following maximums:

	Usual Daily Dosage for Age 65 & Over & Age 12 & Under	**Usual Daily Dosage for Age Under 65 & Over 12**
Ativan	3 mg/day	6 mg/day
Azene	30 mg/day	60 mg/day
Centrax	30 mg/day	60 mg/day
chlordiazepoxide	40 mg/day	100 mg/day
diazepam	20 mg/day	60 mg/day
Equanil	600 mg/day	1600 mg/day
Librium	40 mg/day	100 mg/day
meprobamate	600 mg/day	1600 mg/day
Miltown	600 mg/day	1600 mg/day
Paxipam	80 mg/day	160 mg/day

Serax	60 mg/day	90 mg/day
Valium	20 mg/day	60 mg/day
Tranxene	30 mg/day	60 mg/day
Xanax	2 mg/day	4 mg/day

- More than two changes of an antidepressant within a 7-day period. Examples of commonly used antidepressants are:

	Usual Maximum Daily Dosages for Age 65 & Over	Usual Maximum Daily Dosage
Adapin	150 mg	300 mg
amitriptyline	150 mg	300 mg
Asendin	200 mg	400 mg
Aventyl	75 mg	150 mg
Desyrel	300 mg	600 mg
doxepin	150 mg	300 mg
Elavil	150 mg	300 mg
imipramine	150 mg	300 mg
Ludiomil	150 mg	300 mg
Norpramin	150 mg	300 mg
Pamelor	75 mg	150 mg
Pertofrane	150 mg	300 mg
Sinequan	150 mg	300 mg
SK pramine	150 mg	300 mg
Surmontil	150 mg	300 mg
Tofranil	150 mg	300 mg
Vivacil	30 mg	60 mg

- Use of the antidepressants listed in excess of their listed daily dosage maximums;
- Patients who repeatedly lose seizure control while taking anticonvulsants, e.g., Dilantin (phenytoin), phenobarbital, Mysoline, Depakene (valproic acid);
- Patients who are taking thyroid drugs and have not had some assessment of thyroid function (e.g., Free T4 Level, T3 Resin uptake, Free Thyroid uptake). Examples of commonly used thyroid drugs are Synthroid, Cytomel, Thyroid Extract;
- Patients who are taking the following drugs and have not had a blood pressure recorded at least weekly.

Aldomet	Hylorel
Apresoline	Inderal
Blocadren	Ismelin
Capoten	Lasix
Catapres	Lopressor
chlorothiazide	Minipress
Corgard	propranolol
Diuril	reserpine
Dyazide	Serpasil
furosemide	Tenormin
hydralazine	Visken
hydrochlorothiazide	Wytensin
Hydrodiuril	Zaroxolyn
Hygroton	

- Patients who are taking anticoagulant therapy and have not had some assessment of blood clotting function at least monthly. The most common blood clotting function test is prothrombin time. Examples of commonly used anticoagulants are Coumadin (warfarin), Dicumarol;
- Patients who are taking cardioactive drugs and have not had a pulse rate recorded daily in the first month of therapy and weekly thereafter, *or* the chart shows a pulse consistently below 60 or above 100.

Blocadren	Procan
Calan	Procardia
Corgard	Pronestyl
digoxin	propranolol
Inderal	Quinaglute
Isoptin	quinidine
Lanoxin	Tenormin
Lopressor	Timoptic
Norpace	Visken

- Patients who are taking insulin or oral hypoglycemics and have not had a urine sugar test at least daily *or* a blood sugar test at least every 60 days. Examples of commonly used hypoglycemics are: Glucotrol, Diabeta, Micronase, Orinase, Diabinese, Dymelor, Tolinase;

- Patients who are taking iron preparations, folic acid or vitamin B_{12}, and have not had a red blood cell assessment (e.g., hemoglobin, hematocrit) during the first month of therapy. Examples of commonly used iron preparations are: Feosol (ferrous sulfate), Imferon, Fergon (ferrous gluconate);
- Use of Mandelamine, Hiprex, Bactrim, Septra, Macrodantin, Furadantin, or Urex in chronic urinary tract infections if a urinalysis has not been performed at least once, 30 days after therapy was initiated;
- Patients taking Mandelamine or Hiprex who have not had a urine pH determination within 30 days after therapy was initiated, or if therapy is continued when urine pH is continually above 6;
- Use of nitrofurantoin (Furadantin, Macrodantin) for conditions other than treatment or prophylaxis of urinary tract infections, or blood urea nitrogen or serum creatinine levels are not recorded on the chart;
- Three or more orders for analgesics used at the same time. Examples of commonly used analgesics are:

acetaminophen	Indocin
Anaprox	Meclomen
aspirin	meperidine
Clinoril	Motrine
Darvocet N	Nalfon
Darvon Compound	Naprosyn
Demerol	Percodan
Dolobid	Rufen
Empirin	Tolectin
Empirin with Codeine	Trilisate
Feldene	Tylenol
ibuprofen	Tylenol with Codeine

- Patients taking diuretics who have *not* had a serum potassium level determination within 30 days after initiation of therapy. Examples of commonly used diuretics are:

acetazolamide	Aldactazide
Aldactone	Bumex

chlorothiazide   hydrochlorothiazide
Diamox   Hydrodiuril
Diuril   Hygroton
Dyazide   Lasix
Dyrenium   Midamor
Edecrin   Moduretic
Enduron   Neptazane
Esidrix   Zaroxolyn
furosemide

- Patients taking certain diuretics and cardiotonics, e.g., Lanoxin who have not had a serum potassium determination within 30 days after initiation of the cardiotonic therapy and every 6 months thereafter;
- Patients who are taking Butazolidin, Azolid, or Tandearil continuously and have not had at least one CBC determination 30 days after initiation of therapy;
- The use of cardiotonics, e.g., Lanoxin in the absence of documentation of one of the following diagnoses:
  congestive heart failure
  atrial fibrillation
  paroxysmal supraventricular tachycardia
  atrial flutter
- The use of anticholinergic therapy, e.g., Artane, Cogentin, or Kemadrin with antipsychotic drugs in the absence of recorded extrapyramidal side effects, e.g., tremor, drooling, shuffling gait;
- The continuous use of antibiotic/steroidal opthalmic preparation, e.g., Cortisporin ophthalmic. Metimyd ophthalmic or Ophthocort, for periods exceeding 14 days;
- The use of the following aminoglycosides (Garamycin, Nebcin, Amikin, Kantrex, Netromycin) in the absence of a serum creatinine determination when therapy was initiated;
- Orders for drugs for which there is a known allergy as documented in the patient's record;
- The crushing of solid dosage forms when the likely result will cause patient discomfort (e.g., Dulcolax) or undesired blood levels (e.g., Theo-Dur).

Appendix 15.2 American Society of Consultant Pharmacists Guidelines for Assessing the Quality of Drug Regimen Reviews in Long-term Care Facilities[a]

1. Evaluating Medication Orders: The consultant pharmacist determines whether the resident's medication orders represent optimal therapy for that individual.

2. Monitoring Medication Administration: The consultant pharmacist evaluates medication administration to verify that the resident has received his/her medications in conformance with prescriber's orders and facility policies.

3. Evaluating Response to Drug Therapy: The consultant pharmacist evaluates the resident's response to drug therapy.

4. Communicating Observations and Recommendations: The consultant pharmacist communicates observations and recommendations regarding residents' drug therapy to those with authority and/or responsibility to implement the recommendations and verifies that there has been a response.

5. Supportive Environment: The long-term facility supports pharmacy practices that promote quality care.

[a]Adapted and reprinted with permission from "Guidelines—Assessing the Quality of Drug Regimen Review in Long-term Care Facilities." Copyright © 1989, American Society of Consultant Pharmacists, Inc.

Index

α-Adrenergic agonists, 113, 114
α-Adrenergic blockers, 23–24, 59, 62, 113, 116
α-Blockers, 59, 62
α-Methyldopa, 62
Abdominal infections
  drug therapy, 40–41
  in nursing home patients, 30
Abnormal Involuntary Movement Scale (AIMS), 91
ACE-inhibitors
  in antihypertensive therapy, 59, 61–62
  cardiovascular indications, 122, 127–128
  and renal insufficiency, 20, 121
Acebutolol
  H_2O lipid solubility, 127
  and renal insufficiency, 20
Acetaminophen, 135–136
Acetylcysteine, 135
Achlorhydria, 150, 152
Acidosis, 67
Acute dystonic reactions, 88
Acyclovir, 20
Adalat, 124
Adverse drug effects
  of ACE-inhibitors, 61–62
  of α-methyldopa, 62
  analgesic nephropathy, 136
  of anticholinergic agents, 115
  of antipsychotics, 88–92
  of benzodiazepine, 85
  of β-blockers, 61
  of calcium blockers, 60
  of cardiovascular agents, 122
  central nervous system, 155
  of clonidine, 62
  of diuretics, 60–61
  hyperglycemia, 144
  hypoglycemia, 144
  hypotension, 127
  of NSAIDs, 136

  of opiate antagonists, 137
  of phenytoin, 74–75
  of reserpine, 62
  of sedatives, 22
  sleep disorders, 82
  urinary incontinence, 110
Adverse drug reactions
  and antihypertensive therapy, 56–57
  and complex regimens, 1–3, 9
  depression, 48
  hepatic necrosis, 135
  reporting, 171, 173
  seizures, 67
  and sulfonylurea antihyperglycemics, 145
Aging (*see also* Elderly)
  and adverse drug reactions, 1–2
  and body composition, 14
  and cardiac output, 16–17
  and compliance, 4, 6–9
  and COPD, 158–159
  and diabetes mellitus, 143
  and drug response, 22–25
  gastrointestinal changes in, 12–13
  and serum proteins, 14–16
Agranulocytosis, 92
Akathesia, 90
Albuterol
  and COPD therapy, 158, 159
  and hyperglycemia, 144
Alcohol
  and hypoglycemia, 144
  and peptic disease, 150, 152
  and seizures, 67
Alkalosis, 67
Allopurinol, 20
Alprazolam, 49–51
AlternaGEL, 153
Alupent, 159
Alzheimer's disease, 66
Amantadine, 20

189